The Smart Guide to Infertility

PERSONAL DEDICATIONS

Primary dedication

To Caroline 21.7.1945 - 22.1.2008

My strength and better half, taken too soon

Also

To my children Peta, Sinead, Robert and Charlotte,

my grandchildren

And

To all the one-finger typists everywhere

The Smart Guide to Infertility

myths and reality

By

Professor Robert F Harrison
MA MD DSc FRCS(Ed) FRCOG FRCP(I) DCH

Illustrated and contributed to by the late
Caroline M Harrison

MSc BSS CQSW BASRT(Accred) UKCP IAAAC IACT(Accred)

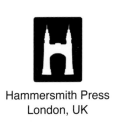

Hammersmith Press
London, UK

First published in 2009 by Hammersmith Press Limited
496 Fulham Palace Road, London, SW6 6JD, UK
www.hammersmithpress.co.uk

Disclaimer
Whilst the advice and information in this book are believed to be true
and accurate at the date of going to press, neither the author nor the
publisher can accept any legal responsibility or liability for any errors or
omissions that may have been made. In particular (but without limiting
the generality of the preceding disclaimer) while every effort has been
made to ensure that the contents of this book are accurate, it must not be
treated as a substitute for qualified medical advice.

British Library Cataloguing in Publication Data: A CIP record of this
book is available from the British Library.

ISBN 978-1-905140-23-7

Commissioning Editor: Georgina Bentliff
Production by Helen Whitehorn, Pathmedia
Designed and typeset by Julie Bennett
Printed and bound by TJ International, Ltd, UK
Cover image: ZenShui / James Hardy / Getty images

Contents

Contents

Contents

Contents

Contents

Acknowledgements

To all the patients and colleagues of all disciplines I have worked for and with over the years. Particular thanks are due to staff in the HARI (Human Assisted Reproduction Ireland) Unit for their support and encouragement and for jogging my memory about techniques when needed. I am also indebted to Dr Cathy Allen, Dr Edgar Mocanu, Mary O'Conor, Anne Marie and Niall Sudway and Kathy and Marcus Cosgrave for putting me right on different issues at the pre-proof stage. I acknowledge being able to quote data from ESHRE, the CDC and HARI. Finally I salute the friendly guidance of Georgina Bentliff of Hammersmith Press who I have found really great at licking the final product into a more user-friendly shape.

About the author and the book

The Author, Robbie Harrison, was brought up in Liverpool, qualifying in Medicine from the Royal College of Surgeons in Ireland (RCSI) Dublin in 1967. He trained in Obstetrics and Gynacology, firstly in Dublin at the Mater and Rotunda Hospitals, moving on in 1972 to Queen Charlotte's and Chelsea Hospitals for Women and The Royal Postgraduate Medical School London University as Lecturer and Honorary Senior Registrar. His in-depth involvement in the management of infertility began then and has continued to the present day, some 37 years later.

Following his return to Dublin in 1976, initially as Consultant/ Senior Lecturer at Trinity College and the Rotunda and then Associate Professor, he set up the first specific, couple-orientated, clinics in Ireland to provide modern management of infertility at the Rotunda and St James's Hospitals. This has included pioneering the various Assisted Reproduction Techniques as they have come on stream clinically, initially at Sir Patrick Dunn's (1985) and St James's (1986) Hospitals, but from 1989 until his retirement from active practice in 2005, back at the Rotunda. It was here where he founded Human Assisted Reproduction Ireland (The HARI Unit) as well as being the Professor and Head of the RCSI Department of Obstetrics and Gynaecology. The Rotunda/HARI Unit services are ongoing and continue to have a worldwide reputation for research, training and couple care and the Unit is the largest and leading provider of these services in the area of Human Reproduction in the Irish Republic.

During his time in Human Reproduction, as befits someone with a worldwide reputation earned through over 210 published peer review papers and 135 invited presentations, amongst honours gained he chaired the WHO Taskforce on Infertility from 1984 to 1988. He was given the Andres Bello First Class Award by the President of Venezuela in 1992 and he served as President of the International Federation of Fertility Societies 1998-2001. In 2008 he became the Irish Fertility Society's first Honorary Fellow.

The Contributor: Throughout this time until her death in January 2008, Robbie's constant companion, muse and mentor was his wife Caroline. Mother to their four children, she was initially a fashion designer, then a social worker and Trinity College Lecturer in Social Studies, becoming latterly the sex and relationship psychotherapist to the Rotunda and HARI unit. She was also a member of the Irish Government Commission on Assisted Human Reproduction (2000-05) and had been steadily gaining recognition as an artist of promise. Now, sadly, written about here posthumously, she is the only other direct contributor to this book. Despite her sudden illness, her qualifications and skills made her the obvious choice to provide the illustrations and the text of the section on 'physical coital problems and sexual dysfunctions'.

This book was written in 2007-8 in the terrible time during the Author's wife's fatal illness with ovarian cancer. It draws foremost upon his experience as a clinician practising daily in the field for over 37 years, but also his knowledge as a teacher, personal researcher and evaluator of the work of others.

He has put together a volume that covers exclusively and comprehensively infertility management as it is today. It is designed principally for those who are wondering if they are infertile. It provides basic facts, personal comments and guidance, but throughout, a greater depth of information is also provided than is perhaps usual in such books as it is this sort of knowledge that, in the Author's experience, the discerning infertile couple of today will demand.

Chapter 1

Objectives

In this guide I aim to provide accurate, up-to-date information on the causes of infertility and on current methods of investigation and treatment. Designed primarily with patients in mind, I hope it may also be useful for healthcare professionals and students occasionally needing in-depth knowledge of the field.

While it should be considered but one of a number of potential sources to be explored, I can confirm that I have written this book in as unbiased a way as possible, drawing on my knowledge and experience in the field, which spans some 37 years. Wherever possible I have included appropriate data from peer-reviewed sources. My personal opinions are summarised and presented clearly as such at the end of each chapter or major chapter-section. I have no commercial affiliations to declare.

The text deliberately introduces the appropriate technical terms that are used by practitioners in the field, together with explanations of each. Simple understandable line drawings and algorithms illustrate salient points. I have described the underlying physiological background (how the body functions) of vital processes, including conception, semen production and the menstrual cycle. It is complex and can be hard to understand; I have tried to simplify it as much as possible but some in-depth knowledge is essential for potentially infertile couples if they are to understand, and cope with, the investigations and treatment that may lie ahead.

My aim is not to replace 'going for appropriate help' with 'DIY', but to provide couples who are finding it difficult to conceive with a framework of general and specific knowledge regarding possible causes, how these are investigated, what the treatment options are, and the chances of success with each so that they can make educated choices through informed discussion with healthcare professionals. For simplicity, when discussing prognosis (the chances of success) related to a specific treatment, I have assumed both partners are normal in all other respects and that the treatment will be carried out fully, as prescribed. This can, of course, give rise to inaccuracy and over- and under-estimations of potential success as there will often be more than one factor involved in infertility. Additionally, the 'fecundability' (probability of conceiving in a single menstrual cycle) or otherwise of the partner not being treated will always play an important part in eventual success, or lack of it.

Understanding what is happening not only is essential for informed consent to any intervention that is proposed, but also optimises the chances of success as knowledge allows couples to become an integral and valued part of the infertility team working on the problem. It also enables patients to evaluate the quality of the service that is being provided. Remember, 'There is more to life and infertility treatment than just IVF!'

Chapter 2

From natural conception to birth

MYTH

Everybody knows and understands how to make babies.

The journey of sperm to oocyte

The most common and natural way of initiating conception is through the act of vaginal intercourse between a man and a woman during the reproductive phases of their lives.

Described in the most simplistic of terms, sperm (more accurately, 'spermatozoa') are released from the male penis at ejaculation into the vagina. They swim up the cervical canal (neck of the womb) into the uterus (womb). From there they enter the two fallopian tubes and pass down to the fimbrial outlets (see Figure 1 on page 5). Leading sperm have been found at the end of the tubes within about 30 minutes.

Approaching the time of ovulation (that is, the time once every 28 days when a woman releases an egg), the end of each fallopian tube moves nearer its adjacent ovary. Sperm either meet the egg (or ovum) just inside the tube whose fimbrial processes have 'hoovered' it up or exit the tube to meet the ovum just outside. If ovulation has not yet taken place, the sperm can live in the woman for up to three days but the egg is only viable and sufficiently mature for fertilisation for 12 hours.

Fertilisation

Fertilisation is the name of a process whereby two gametes (a sperm and an egg) fuse together to create a new individual with genetic potential derived from both parents. It is a very complex process that will take place only if a sperm enters the egg; it is not a fixed single event occurring in one moment of time but takes 20 to 30 hours.

The nucleus of every human cell contains 46 chromosomes, arranged in 23 pairs, which in turn contain all the genetic coding necessary for human cells to develop. However, the nuclei of the gametes (the egg and the sperm) each contain only 23 unpaired chromosomes, reduced to this number by a process called 'meiosis'.

Eggs develop from cells called 'primary oocytes' present in the woman's ovaries from way before birth. Meiosis produces a secondary oocyte (cell with potential to become an egg) with 23 chromosomes while the unneeded 23 are expelled from the cell in something called the 'first polar body'. Once the 'secondary oocyte' (we will now call it the 'egg') has been released by its ovary, it is mature and begins to divide for a second time but this process is completed only when activated by the entry of a sperm into the egg. The egg nucleus, called the 'pronucleus', continues to have 23 chromosomes, including the female sex chromosome denoted as X. The other 23 non-used chromosomes produced by the second division of the egg are expelled from the fertilising cell as something called the 'second polar body'.

Development of the sperm also involves meiosis, producing a nucleus containing again 23 chromosomes including the sex chromosome. In this case, because men have the sex chromosome configuration XY, it can be either a female (X) chromosome or a male (Y) chromosome, which in turn will determine the gender of the offspring. Sperm then undergo a process known as activation and capacitation, that takes place over some hours. This is necessary if a sperm is to penetrate the outer skin of the egg (zona pellucida).

If a sperm succeeds in entering the egg, its tail detaches itself and degenerates. Meanwhile, its pronucleus, which forms the swollen head of the mature sperm, migrates to the centre of the egg to make contact with the female pronucleus. The two pronuclei align and fuse. This process is called 'syngamy'.

The 23 egg chromosomes pair up with the 23 sperm chromosomes to form a cell (known as a zygote) that has the normal chromosomal content of all other body cells – that is, 46, including two sex cells. These may be XX, denoting the offspring is female, if an X-carrying sperm fertilised the egg, or XY (male offspring) if a Y-carrying sperm got there first.

Figure 1 Schematic diagram of conceptual events

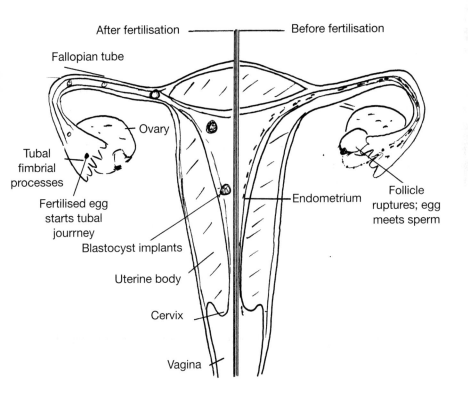

Development of the embryo before it reaches the uterus

Rapid cell division, or 'reduplication', then commences, the zygote initially dividing into two identical cells, around 36 hours after insemination. (Cell division is by a process called 'mitosis' which involves the complete replication of all 46 chromosomes in the cell, and is the process by which all cell division in the body associated with growth and repair takes place.) Two then divide to become four after 40 hours, then eight, then sixteen, and so on over the next few days while the fertilised egg is still in the fallopian tube. Up until there are eight cells, this is under maternal genetic control; thereafter, development becomes self-determined. The cells formed at this stage are what is known as 'totipotent', meaning that any single one is capable of forming any type of cell.

What were initially identical cells (blastomeres) begin to differentiate until by four to five days after fertilisation the zygote has grown to become a 'blastocyst', with a fluid-filled cavity surrounded by two layers of cells. One layer is called the 'inner cell mass'. This is destined to give rise to the tissues which will form the embryo, and eventually the baby, once the blastocyst has become implanted in the wall of the uterus. The other, outer, layer will form the 'extra embryonic tissue' which is involved in the formation of the placenta. The cells have now instead become 'pluripotent'. This means that they are capable of forming different parts/structures of the embryo. This is the stage desired by those who wish to develop stem cell cultures from embryonic cells and hopefully generate new tissues where organ failure has occurred. The uterine cavity is reached by the blastocyst stage embryo at 5–6 days post insemination. It is still inside its surrounding 'skin' or zona pellucida.

Development of the embryo within the uterus

For the healthy development of the embryo, the blastocyst needs to be implanted into the lining of the wall of the uterus, otherwise known as the endometrium. However, this does not happen as soon as the blastocyst arrives in the uterus as it first has to 'hatch'. This happens on the 7th or 8th day, when the outer layer or 'zona pellucida' ruptures. Then the hormone, human chorionic gonadotrophin (hCG), starts to be produced and by day 11-12 the further developing blastocyst is fully implanted.

Early tissue development (gastrulation) commences about day 14 and the 'primitive streak', which is the first sign of the head to toe axis of the embryo, is formed at this time. Blood starts to flow through the placental system and circulation is established. The initial differentiation of the embryo's organs (organogenesis) continues for some eight weeks. Embryo cell formation is likely to be complete by 12 weeks, the majority of cells now being able only to reproduce their own kind – that is, they are now 'unipotent'.

Fetal life up until birth

Nourished by the mother via the placenta, the embryo and its organs continue to grow, becoming what is known by eight weeks as the fetus. Birth and the beginning of independent life should occur at approximately 280 days.

* * *

Personal Comment

Misconceptions about the processes of reproduction abound; I hope this chapter will have given you a clear picture.

You will see there is no single fixed point that can be identified as the exact beginning of independent human life, though truly independent life actually only begins at birth. Interpretation of the facts as to when 'life begins' varies. Initial cell development is controlled by the mother until the

6-8 cell stage, but then switches to self-determination with some paternal genome influence. However, without implantation in the uterine wall the potential that exists in this group of live cells cannot ever be actualised. I share my medico-moral position on the pre-implantation embryo with the American Society for Reproductive Medicine who in 2004 stated, 'although because of its potential, the human embryo from fertilization is worthy of special respect, it does not have the status to be entitled to the same rights and protection as a person.'

Chapter 3

What is infertility and who may it affect?

MYTH

Infertility is rare and unlikely to happen to me – or us.

Definition

The World Health Organisation (WHO) defined infertility in 2001 as 'failure to conceive after at least one year of unprotected intercourse'. It may be primary, when no conception has ever occurred, or secondary, when there has been a conception in the past even if a baby was not the final result.

Data shows that 80% or so of couples having regular normal intercourse successfully conceive during that first year of trying and 70% take home a baby. Indeed, of those remaining, another 50% will conceive naturally in the next year, 40% or so with a live birth. These chances drop as female age increases and time goes on, but during the reproductive phase of life, except in the absence of vital organs of reproduction and with the possible exceptions of totally blocked tubes or no sperm, it is foolhardy and wrong to say that a couple have no chance of natural conception ever, no matter how slim it may be.

Some couples seem to be able to plan when to conceive and just do; others, often to their surprise, cannot. It can happen to anyone. Whether a couple conceive together or not depends on adding together the fertility potential of both partners. High potential in one can compensate for lower potential in the other; a minor problem in one partner may therefore never come to light if the other has high fertility potential. Infertility is a couple's problem and should always be approached and treated as such.

When to suspect there may be a problem

The definition suggests that a couple should wait at least one year before seeking help and if young (under 30) maybe up to two years to allow nature to take its course. However, previous illnesses may lead people to suspect they may have difficulty in conceiving earlier than this. If either or both of you are really worried, although DIY home kits can be used to 'check' both your semen quality and ovulation, it is best that you seek the advice of your doctor early on. You should also do so if you have coital problems or infrequent periods.

Time can be important. A woman's fertility decreases with age. Her chances of conceiving reduce from 74% to 54% at 35+ years, and the risk of fetal abnormality and abortion increases from 10% when she is under 30 to 34% when 40+. If the woman is over 35 years of age, it is advisable to wait no longer than six months before commencing investigations. The so-called male 'amber light' starts at 40.

Incidence

Sub-fertility can be considered a fairly common problem. It is thought that up to one in six to one in eight of couples (15%) may have difficulties in conceiving. This is predicted to increase in the future as more people postpone pregnancy on economic grounds. In Australia, for instance, in the last 30 years the number of women conceiving their first child under 30 years of age has dropped from 92% to 27%, with a stable relationship and a good income being cited as more important before starting a family than partner age. Indeed, less than half knew that the woman's age was a factor in determining their chances of conceiving.

Causes

Causes vary in different parts of the world. The potential problem may be detected on the male side in some 30% of cases and on the female in approximately 50%. In 10%, both partners may have a problem, but in up to 20% no cause is found.

This latter situation is then generally labelled 'Unexplained Infertility', meaning simply that no cause has been found (see chapter 10, page 173), currently available tests not being able to detect what could be going wrong.

Secondary infertility

Secondary infertility is a surprisingly common finding in both general-infertility and IVF clinics, with some 25-30% and 30-32% of couples respectively having at least one partner who has already had at least one conception. For one reason or another, not all these past conceptions will have been successful and they may still be childless (chapter 10, pages 182-93). Also circumstances may lead to a child not always being brought up by the birth mother or father.

Secondary infertility is thought to be on the increase. Couples often delay having further children for social reasons, so the age of attempting conception goes up. Likewise, a change of partner may be the reason for someone attempting to conceive again. This is a major reason nowadays as so many relationships seem to break down.

If you are amongst those within the definition of 'secondary infertility', you have possible advantages over those with primary in-fertility in that where a couple have conceived together previously, the prognosis for further conception has been found to be better – that is, nearly twice as high as where the partnership is now different and one third better compared with a couple with primary infertility. Additionally, when investigations are contemplated, your past reproductive history may also help the infertility team target potential causes for your present childlessness.

Couples with secondary infertility should expect to be treated in the same way as if they had primary infertility in terms of criteria for intervention and mode of management and support.

Personal Comment

Childlessness has no boundaries. Recommendations as to the optimum time to seek help are based on natural conceptions and may not be right for the individual case. They may work in a couple's best interests by preventing an unnecessarily early referral and intervention but I feel that individual circumstances should dictate. Couples may become anxious if they do not conceive immediately after starting to try. This may be counter-productive and premature, but waiting excessively long before seeking out possible causes may bring female age into the equation. This cannot be emphasised too often. And for this reason, conception the second time around may not be so easy as the first. Whether or not a child has already been born to one or other partner or the couple together, it is a legitimate desire to want more; I consider that, with few exceptions, this aspiration too is fully deserving of medical support.

Chapter 4

Things to think about before seeking help

MYTH

Everybody wants children!

Is the time right?

If you are wondering if you have a fertility problem, before seeking any help, the most important factor that needs to be discussed and agreed upon is that having a child at this time is what both of you truly desire. As a couple you may be embarking on what can be a long, stressful journey, sometimes with great rewards at the end, but sometimes not.

Secondary to this agreement is that when seeking help you both agree on how far and for how long you wish to take treatment. This is important as some relationships will blossom in this situation and a couple become closer, but, in others, the cracks soon begin to show. This is especially true if one partner is being pressurised into doing something they really do not wish to do at this time. Many can feel mistakenly that having a baby will restore a broken relationship but this is not the right motive and it seldom works!

If, as a couple, you decide to go ahead, at all consultations, whatever investigation or treatment is suggested, it is vital to clarify all negatives and weigh them up against the positives before agreeing to participate.

If the positives win then by all means proceed, but if not, do not. This is because infertility, unlike some other medical situations, is not usually life-threatening but, as with all medicine, investigations and treatment can cause health problems (morbidity) and, rarely, death (mortality). Such problems are usually minimised in infertility by patients generally being in good health at the start of the process. However, if you think the risks of damaging your health are too great or if after starting everything becomes too much, stop!

Lifestyle

Modern urban living has brought benefits to many of us in terms of standards of living. Many of the diseases associated with poverty, at least in the western world, are not the common threat they once were. This has not, however, been without cost. This may affect conceptual chances and some diseases have been replaced by others that can reduce fertility.

In order to maintain accustomed lifestyles, demanding work-schedules are often necessary for both partners. Leisure time spent together becomes minimised.

This can be compounded by the need to commute long distances or even live apart for much of the week. Fatigue and stress (see chapter 10, pages 164-72) set in and you, the couple, literally find yourselves too tired to make love as often as you should or would wish to. Consequently, although by definition (chapter 3, page 9), this is not truly infertility, conception does not happen. Such lifestyle is commonplace nowadays in many countries. It is no wonder that in many EU countries there are declining fertility rates.

In such circumstances a reassessment of lifestyle is essential. It may be possible to alter goals and circumstances somewhat, but one partner giving up their job even if it were practical is not usually the solution. Indeed, for you, there may not be one.

Health and wellbeing

Throughout life, but especially as age progresses, regular general health checks for all males and females are advisable through your family practitioner. In infertility, as the potential carrier of a future child, the emphasis rightly or wrongly is on the female. Regular breast checks and cervical smears are advisable as part of keeping all women well. Before embarking on pregnancy, a woman should make sure she is rubella immune. If not, vaccination should be carried out first as rubella infection can pass on to the embryo or fetus and lead to severe congenital malformations.

Diet

Advice abounds from many differing sources, selling the benefits of a good healthy diet for both men and women from a basic health viewpoint. Many 'experts' go further, suggesting that adding a particular supplement or product to a person's diet will help prevent some specific disease or enhance the chances of treatment success. Couples who wish to conceive are not immune to what is often unsubstantiated hard-sell (chapter 12, pages 247-51). However, it is undoubtedly true that if you have a good, balanced, regularly consumed diet without excess, this does help general health and cannot hinder the chances of conception.

All women wishing to conceive should start a regular daily dose of folic acid (400 micrograms) plus vitamin B_{12} as this helps prevent neural tube defects in a baby and some feel may help prevent miscarriages. No more than four units of alcohol should be drunk per week. A 2009-published UK study has shown only 3% of women comply.

Weight

This is the time for both of you to evaluate as truthfully and realistically as you can any potential weight problems. This can be either one or both of you being underweight or, more particularly, overweight. A couple need to consider whether this could be a possible contributing factor that requires attention. It is more likely to contribute directly to infertility in women than in men.

The measure used universally for adults is the Body Mass Index (BMI). It is calculated from a person's weight in kilograms divided by his/her height in metres squared – for example, weight 70 kg divided by height 1.75 m squared, that is 70 divided by 1.75 x 1.75 = BMI 22.9. The healthy range is considered to be 18.5-24.9, overweight to be 25-29.9 and obesity to be 30+ (very, 40+) (World Health Organisation).

Underweight

If an adult woman is underweight (BMI <18.4), this may affect her genital tract organ development and ovulation. This can occur with anorexia nervosa or bulimia. The effects on the reproductive organs' size are usually reversible with appropriate treatment, but anorexia and bulimia are serious and difficult diseases to treat that need attention first and mortality is not unknown.

Being overweight for height

You are overweight for height when you have a Body Mass Index (BMI) of 25-29.9. In a woman this can be associated with ovulation problems such as occur in the polycystic ovarian syndrome (PCOs) (see page 129). As an overweight woman's BMI increases, there is a 4% drop in her fertility for every unit rise between 30 and 35. Where her BMI is over 35, she is between 26% and 49% less likely to conceive compared with women with a BMI in the normal range.

In men, semen and coital function may be adversely affected, either directly or through a tendency towards diabetes.

If you are overweight, individually or as a couple, a truthful personal approach to a self-regulating diet and calorie intake plus exercise may be enough to alleviate the situation and allow normality to be restored. If you are an obese man or woman with a BMI of 30+ (a BMI of 30 indicates excess body weight of 30%) and, in particular, if you are morbidly obese for your height, pre-conceptual attention to weight is essential. This is not only to aid conception but more especially for general health reasons. Indeed, for safety some clinics will demand a specifically targeted weight reduction, especially in the woman, prior to initiating investigations or treatment.

If you recognise that you have a weight problem and self-help has not apparently worked, now may be the ideal time to seek advice from a dietician or a group such as Weight Watchers from a general health as well as a fertility point of view.

Where weight problems are excessive, the solution is unlikely to be simple. A multi-disciplinary approach to what is usually a multi-factorial (many interrelated causes) situation is likely to be required at a specialised weight-loss clinic. Diet is needed but you must maintain losses. The goal of having a baby can be great motivation but behavioural modification may be needed. If you are morbidly obese, lipase (fat) inhibitor drugs such as orlistat, and operations such as gastric stapling or banding, may also need to be considered.

Addictions

Alcohol and the use of street drugs (chapters 7 and 9, pages 43 and 112) such as marijuana, cocaine, or heroin, may all contribute to infertility by inhibiting gonadal function and thus sperm and egg production. The lifestyle that goes with addiction is not the environment in which to bring up a child. An in-recovery situation needs to be achieved first.

While excessive consumption of alcohol and cigarette smoking by either or both partners has been linked to decreased fecundity, ceasing such practices is certainly also conducive to better overall health. This is not just for the sake of the couple themselves but also the fetus in utero. There is strong evidence of the undesirable effects these substances can have in utero, which can carry through into post-delivery development.

The cost – outlay of money and time

In addition to the unmeasurable potential cost of stress to everyday life that couples may feel when going for help (chapter 10, pages 164-72), you must understand that there are inevitable concrete costs involved for everybody. These include your time and money, even if clinic attendance and the procedures carried out and drugs prescribed are covered by insurance or the NHS. This is particularly true of the Assisted Reproduction Technique (ART) group of therapies (chapter 11, pages 194-246).

Circumstances differ from country to country and, sometimes in areas within them. Couples must make enquiries as to what the outlay is likely to be. This is essential to avoid misunderstandings later on. It must be understood that if you are opting for the private sector, charges will be levied for everything. You will need to explore with the clinic before the first consultation the potential costs involved. It is wise to obtain a reasonable item-by-item estimate of likely costs. This should be possible for the basic profile of investigations and certain procedures, but no clinic will be able to foresee how far things may have to be taken.

You should construct an affordable budget but it is wise for couples to set aside extra contingency funds. No one should get into serious debt to go privately. Better to opt for public healthcare than this if possible!

For couples with private insurance cover, the wise check eligibility for infertility treatment and what is/is not covered. Different schemes behave differently. Not all the financial outlay will be directly clinical or medical in origin. There are hidden costs that also need to be contemplated, which, if forgotten, may be difficult to cope with.

Whether public or private, some financial expenses will inevitably occur, to be borne totally from your own pockets. The cost of such items as travel, parking, accommodation, food, and phone calls, child- and dog-minding when attending the clinic/hospital can add up to a considerable sum of money over the time of attendance.

There is very little written about this in any country, but recently published research figures from my own clinic in Ireland estimate the average hidden costs at between €104 and €703 for a typical IVF cycle. These will vary depending on the number of attendances and by whom, and the distance travelled each time. Living near to the clinic is a distinct advantage and will minimise such extras but not eliminate them (chapter 11, pages 213-14).

The biggest potential hidden expense is, however, time off work due to travel for attendance at the clinic. Loss of earnings may need to be factored into the hidden expense calculations. While in this very private situation, many of you may not want to admit to your employers that one or both of you needs time off for infertility treatment, disclosure may lead to surprising co-operation and understanding. This is the wisest route to take as it is not always possible to predict when time off is needed or how long to allow when taking statutory leave or holidays.

During the same IVF cycles quoted above (minimum seven visits), the women on average spent between 35 and 75 hours off work and between 15 and 139 hours travelling, depending on their distance from the hospital. These figures will of course probably double if their partners support them by attending each time.

While many couples might prefer the anonymity of a clinic that is a distance away from where they live, or about which extraordinary claims of successes have been made, there is a distinct advantage to staying as near home as possible. It is also potentially less stressful.

Personal Comment

For most couples, having a child is a major part of their future together. Some will stop at nothing to achieve that aim. Not all share that view. The pressures of society can dominate, but it is important to be sure right at the start that a child is really what you want. Children must always be wanted.

The decision to remain childless, either for the present or forever, is equally valid. I feel strongly that it is wrong to embark on investigations and treatment prematurely, or when the couple are not in agreement.

Anxiety can make a couple vulnerable to exploitation. Realism about your personal circumstances and budget following careful research in this area by yourselves is as essential as prior realistic appraisal of lifestyle, health and body weight.

I consider the potential child's welfare to be paramount. Be aware of the consequences of the use and abuse of drugs with potentially undesirable effects and the need to stop indulging in them if a child is to be given the best chance of fulfilling his or her potential from the time of conception.

Chapter 5

When and where to seek help

MYTH

Go to the best known, maximum publicity-seeking clinic. They must have the best results!

The general (primary care) practitioner

The first port of call should always be your general practitioner (GP). Prior warning to the doctor as to what the consultation is all about is important, as you will find that such consultations take time. This will be especially true if your doctor has an interest in fertility and, rather than just providing a referral letter to a hospital, wishes to give some basic advice and perform some preliminary investigations first.

As with any medical consultation anywhere, it will benefit you to sit down beforehand and discuss issues between yourselves. Write down a check-list of what you want to cover, and the questions you want answered. This will help to give structure to the consultation and may prevent after-thoughts that come to mind too late, after the meeting has finished.

Some investigations and treatments can have significant side effects. It is well worth enquiring about potential risks and costs. Knowledge of your personal circumstances will also allow the GP to give advice about where best to go for specialist treatment and whether this should be state-funded or private (see chapter 4, pages 18-19).

The initial consultation at the GP surgery

Infertility is a couple's problem. Both you and your partner need to be there for the initial consultation and also throughout any further meetings wherever possible. Fault is not what this is about.

As with any doctor/patient first consultation, you should expect this first meeting to include a full medical history of both you and your partner. You may find this quite probing, comprehensively covering your whole life to date. The patient's history is the most vital part of any consultation and is used by the doctor to decide the way to go. While the discussion itself may range around many issues and appear unstructured at times, so as to miss nothing out, all doctors are trained to record what is said in a specific way under certain headings. In infertility, history taking differs from most situations as a couple are involved. Both of you will be questioned and your answers recorded separately.

These will start with the 'the presenting complaint', which is briefly what you are coming to the doctor for recorded in your own words. A 'history of the presenting complaint' is then written down from your answers to the doctor's questions. A full 'past history' of any illnesses will be taken and recorded as will a full, relevant 'family medical history' and your 'social histories'. Finally, both of you will be taken through a 'review of your body systems'. In infertility, the doctor will want to know, for example, the woman's rubella and cervical smear status, and whether she is taking folic acid (see chapter 4, page 15).

Depending on the 'presenting complaint', different specific questions of relevance will be posed. In particular, the doctor needs to check and decide that you as a couple are really infertile, that you know enough about the fertile time in the monthly cycle and that you are having appropriate, regular sex (see chapter 6, page 29). If these criteria are satisfied, the consultation can move on to the key issue: 'Do you wish anything to be done about the problem and if so what?'

In order to answer this key question you will need to be given an outline of the tests that are usually performed to find out what is going wrong (see chapter 6) and to understand that these investigations cannot show everything. Equally, they may show that the underlying problem is one for which there is no active treatment available. The treatment that is used may fail and IVF is not necessarily the appropriate first, or final, resort in your situation despite what you may have thought. If you wish to go ahead on this understanding, the doctor can then proceed to examine you both physically and set the next investigatory steps in motion.

In a number of instances such potentially reassuring measures are sufficient and conception spontaneously occurs before a decision to refer on for further investigation and treatment is deemed necessary. This is an example of the positive placebo effect, a well-recognised occurrence in infertility (see end of this chapter, page 26).

In the primary care/GP setting, if, instead of taking a detailed history at your first visit, your doctor refers you to a hospital straight away, you may find that no relevant intimate examinations are carried out apart from a general systems review.

Where the GP does refer you on, his/her backing and support later on can prove of great assistance to all concerned and an essential aid to the endeavours of the infertility clinic's team on your behalf.

Initial DIY measures

You may already be aware that DIY kits are available to check the man's semen. They stain sperm and give different colours above and below counts of 20 million or supply a microscope so you can count the sperm yourself. Indeed, you may have already attempted this. However, it is generally more informative to ask your GP to arrange for a formal semen analysis. This can usually be ordered locally.

Similarly, you may already be aware how women can make basic checks for ovulation from their menstrual history, physical vaginal mucus signs and temperature charts (see chapter 9, pages 111-18). Again, you may already be doing this. If not, no matter, for taking basal body temperature (BBT) charts unsupervised over a long period of time is potentially stressful and therefore not to be recommended. However, your doctor may perhaps ask you to chart a cycle or two of BBT charts (see Figure 11, page 117) and maybe include cervical mucus changes (Figure 10, page 111) to help optimise coital timing. Again, kits are now available over the counter, using urine or saliva, to detect the woman's most fertile time, but to take any such measures for too long may become very stressful and can lead to coital difficulties (chapter 10, page 165) and failure to ovulate (anovulation) (see chapter 9, page 116).

The general gynaecologist/urologist (secondary care)

In what is generally the next step in infertility and is termed the 'secondary care setting', couples can expect investigations and treatment options to follow many of those delineated below in the chapters to come. Not all will need to go on to have tertiary care. Whatever hospital you attend, all gynaecological consultants will have received basic training in aspects of male and female human reproduction, as will urologists to whom a potential male problem may be referred.

Excellent results can be obtained in the secondary care setting in terms of diagnosis and treatment for couples whose histories indicate this is the appropriate level of care provided the unit concerned has the appropriate expertise and background facilities. Insufficiently up-to-date training or back-up facilities may render the use of some procedures inappropriate and unsafe at this level.

When the limits of local care have been reached or what has been attempted has failed, referral on to a tertiary care centre for further help is wise. This is especially true where advanced investigations and treatments are needed, including therapies such as many types of assisted reproduction technique (ART) (see chapter 11, pages 194-246), gonadotrophin ovulation induction (see chapter 9, page 124) and major reproductive surgery (see chapters 7 and 8, pages 55, 72, and 101). Indeed, your GP may think the tertiary care centre should in fact be the initial port of call if you are already living in its catchment area.

Tertiary care

In a true tertiary care centre, you can expect to find an appropriately qualified, experienced and dedicated team of trained doctors, laboratory staff, nurses, counsellors and administrators working in surroundings aimed at providing a comprehensive gold standard of care in any required area for any infertile attendees.

In some centres, tertiary care is mainly dedicated to the provision of types of ART (assisted reproductive techniques) (see chapter 11, pages 194-246). In others, some form of ART will still be the main aspect of treatment offered but not the whole. If you and your GP think you need the full gamut of investigations and possible treatments, it is important to ensure the centre to which you are referred can offer what you need. Be sure that expert counselling is available to help throughout but especially should you decide at any time to call a halt (counselling-out).

If you are unhappy with what one tertiary care centre can or has done for you, you may benefit from a second opinion even at this specialised level of care. But going from clinic to clinic or doctor to doctor in an endless search for what may be impossible to achieve is not recommended. No matter what claims are made, no one unit or person has the monopoly on success.

Some tertiary care units are free-standing and at a distance from general hospital services. It is worth checking in these circumstances that access to in-patient hospital facilities will be available to cope with any complications. There should also be appropriate liaison with the couple's chosen maternity unit if they are successful.

No shows

Whatever the setting, primary, secondary or tertiary, if you are unable to keep an appointment, please, please cancel in good time. Someone else can then be given the slot. No shows are a serious problem, particularly for a first visit. At my own state-funded clinic we found that nearly one third (32%) of appointments were not kept, 23% without warning, compared with 17% of those attending privately with only 2% non-notified. This tallies with general reports. In some cases this may have been because the woman had become pregnant in the mean time (a long-distance placebo effect); it is true that where hospitals have poor communication systems the act of cancellation can be made so difficult patients eventually give up trying.

The 'placebo effect'

There is a background level of natural conception, as also explained in chapter 3 (see pages 9-10). In the first year of trying, up to 80% of couples will conceive, with 70% having a live birth. A further 50% of those left will conceive in the second year. This proportion decreases with rising female age but, unless there are insuperable barriers, in the majority of couples the chances of having a baby never disappears completely between the menarche (start of periods) and the menopausal years. However, as the time waiting to conceive goes on and the woman's age rises, this chance does get very low and any conception will come as an 'out of the blue' surprise.

To this baseline level of conception, credit for achieving a pregnancy may also have to be given to the impact attending for help itself seems to have. 'No active treatment was being used at the time of conception,' is therefore always in the background in infertility. It works in favour of the couple throughout all infertility consultations, investigations and treatments.

Recent research, albeit not on infertile couples but on women labelled as having irritable bowel syndrome, has shown that being on the waiting list does improve clinical symptoms, as does being given a placebo. However, having a supportive patient-practitioner relationship seems to exert the most important placebo-type of influence. In infertility, this placebo effect is the control background success rate against which the efficacy of any active treatment should, if at all possible, be judged.

Excluding people with absent vital body structures, no sperm or totally blocked tubes, in my experience a proportion of couples presenting for help can expect to conceive spontaneously, some even by the time of the first visit (2%), and in the days before IVF, I found some 48% conceived during a cycle in which they did not receive active therapy.

Data, both controlled and uncontrolled, suggest the placebo effect gives rise to at least 20-30% of all conceptions occurring within one year in hitherto infertile couples, especially those with mild male or mild ovulation factors and unexplained infertility (see chapters 7, 9 and 10). It is still noted to occur even where couples are listed for IVF, the therapy that is invariably the end of the line. I have reported that between 11% and 16% of couples may conceive before the cycle of IVF treatment starts and, after a couple with unexplained infertility have been successful with IVF, 21% have been shown to conceive again without help within two years.

Personal Comment

Much can be achieved initially together and with the help of your GP, without going near a hospital. Taking the first step at the right time is important, whether this results in the appropriate treatment or triggers that so important, potentially positive, placebo effect whose presence should always be acknowledged.

Clinic self-publicity and league tables may be misleading. Couples can be so desperate that they are easily exploited in the pursuit of their goal. Professional advice from those who should know your circumstances is essential to avoid this happening. A well-informed GP is best and not the internet, books, TV, newspaper headlines, magazine articles or acquaintances met on public transport, at work or anywhere else.

Chapter 6

Investigation at the clinic

MYTH

The hospital clinic will always find out what is wrong and correct it.

First consultation – basic aims

To have a good relationship with your doctor and other clinic members is essential. It will help your participation as part of the infertility team become a reality.

An advance insight into what is likely to be encountered at your first visit will help build this relationship.

It is important for you to try to ensure that the aims of the medical team helping you coincide with your own. It is also important that you clarify right from the start what the aims are and how you might wish these to be achieved. In partnership with yourselves, the main aim of the infertility clinic should be to define the cause of infertility and alleviate it if at all possible and, in addition, to ensure the safety and continuity of any pregnancies that you may have during the time under their care. The clinic should also aim to be able to bring you through to a final resolution if you do not manage to conceive.

History taking

After the initial introductions, you will invariably find that a full history of both of you will be taken, similar to that taken in the primary care setting by your GP (chapter 5, pages 21-3). This, as I have said already, is the foundation for all subsequent consultations, investigations and treatments. You will find that in whatever level of clinic, the format will be similar, but with the underlying benefit of a good referral letter from your GP, a more focused and in-depth approach can be taken immediately.

You will usually find that your description of the 'presenting complaint' (infertility) and your 'medical histories', both present and past, are dealt with first. You will be asked about your ages, length of infertility, present or past diseases and therapies and, if you are secondarily infertile, any information concerning past pregnancies. Indeed, anything that could impact on your fertility or health in general will be questioned. You will both be asked about your psycho-sexual history, including frequency of intercourse.

Family histories will concentrate on familial and hereditary diseases that the extended family may have had in the past or present that might affect either of you or a baby later on. Social and cultural histories are particularly important to explore. Some occupations may be significant, and your domestic living arrangements either together or separately may be the root cause of the problem. Distances to travel for help can cause you significant logistical problems affecting investigation and conception chances. You will both be asked about your smoking and drinking habits and drugs used past and present, prescribed and 'recreational'.

Physical examination

You should both be prepared for a full physical examination. Its timing and extent will depend in part on what is deemed appropriate on the basis of the history you have given and the results of any tests already carried out. At the least, however, examinations are likely to include overall general physical assessment and, in particular, relevant cardio-vascular (blood pressure, pulse rate and heart sounds), respiratory (listen to the lungs), and basic nervous system examinations.

As a woman, you will find that a full breast and gynaecological examination will only usually be performed at an appropriate non-menstruating time in a cycle. This is usually preceded by a methodical examination of the abdomen with you lying on your back on a couch or gynaecological chair. This allows the examiner access to the vagina and, with the help of the left hand on your abdomen, to perform a bimanual examination. The site and size of the pelvic organs can be assessed by the finger inserted into the vagina up as far as the cervix. A metal or plastic instrument called a speculum can also be used to open the vaginal walls to visualise the cervix. This will allow a smear and a post-

Figure 2 Vaginal speculum (duckbill type)

Made of stainless steel (reusable) or plastic (disposable)

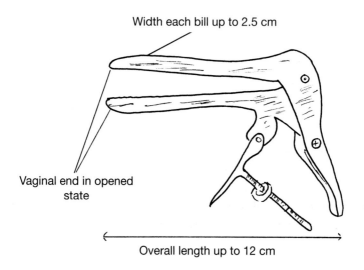

Width each bill up to 2.5 cm

Vaginal end in opened state

Overall length up to 12 cm

coital test, if scheduled (see chapter 10, pages 136-44), to be taken.

As a male, unlike your partner for whom genital tract examination is inevitable, while such a full physical examination is actually just as appropriate, regrettably in this imperfect world it is usually only performed where your history demands it or if any problems with your semen have been suspected or found. Such a male genital examination will be conducted with you standing up and include specifically a check for over-tight underwear. Your penis and scrotal contents will be checked, particularly the testicular size and the possible presence of a varicocele (a varicose vein next to the testicle). A rectal examination may also sometimes be carried out.

Plan of action towards investigation and possible treatment

Before the end of the first consultation a plan of campaign can be formulated between the doctor and yourselves. If needed, changes in lifestyle, weight management and stress will usually be discussed with you at this stage. You will find it helpful if you are given an outline of what tests and treatments are available and can be expected in your own case.

How this is achieved above and beyond history taking and physical examination through to specific investigations may differ in some couples and between clinics. It will be dependent on the context in which help is being sought and in addition be tempered by the interest, training and facilities available and whether the setting is secondary or tertiary (see chapter 5, pages 24-5).

The optimal way forward for all infertile couples is for the clinic to investigate as fully as is possible, in an orderly, organised, routine manner, the main regions that are vital to success (see overleaf, the fertility profile, and chapters 7-10). This should be completed before any treatment (if any) is contemplated. In planning the process of investigation and treatment, you must feel that you are fully engaged, and participatory. It is, however, very important that you understand that as it is the

Figure 3 Fertility profile and basic test used for each region

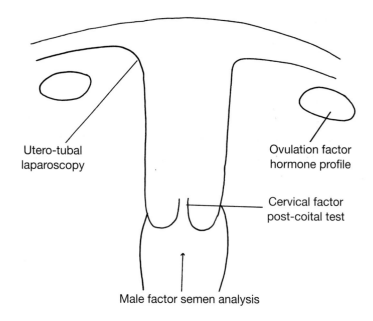

Utero-tubal
laparoscopy

Ovulation factor
hormone profile

Cervical factor
post-coital test

Male factor semen analysis

human condition that is under scrutiny, there are constraints and results cannot be guaranteed to be exact. You may find tests need to be repeated and that results are subject to error.

Quite often (up to 20%) nothing is found. Such couples are labelled as having 'unexplained infertililty' simply due to the imperfections of the investigations that are available today (see chapter 10, pages 173-82).

The 'fertility profile'

A doctor's approach to solving any problem for a patient, including infertility, depends on obtaining clues to the cause from the history followed by a physical examination and, where necessary, further specific investigations. It is hoped this will identify the reason(s) for the problem and the prognosis (chances of the problem being overcome) through to selecting possible suitable therapies.

Chapter 6

How infertility problems are investigated and treated is most conveniently understood if the process is divided according to the four basic regions (see Figure 3, page 32) that make up what I call the 'fertility profile'. There is no true specific order in which tests in these regions should be carried out, although the less invasive tests come first, especially semen analysis.

I have listed the regions here in the order of a sperm's progress towards the egg. First there is the male himself. Then comes the cervical region in the woman. The utero-tubal region, which includes the uterus, tubes and the nearby peritoneum, is next, with ovulation, the final goal for the sperm, last. Together these make up the 'fertility profile' (see also chapter 2, page 3).

In each region, as chapters 7-10 discuss, a single specific test can generally be used to determine in general terms whether a potential causative factor of infertility may exist in that region. The four initial basic tests, in my opinion, are: semen analysis, the post-coital test (PCT), hormonal ovulation tests, and a test of tubal function, preferably by laparoscopy (see chapter 8, pages 82-3).

However, these regions are wide, most covering more than one area of the body, and therefore, as can happen in the overall profile, in themselves they may also contain more than one potential problem. When a specific region appears to be involved, then further and perhaps more costly and invasive tests can be carried out to try to clarify the cause definitively.

Although this recommended approach is not followed specifically, or in all its facets, by all practitioners in the area of infertility it is arguably the most cost-effective, quickest and most comprehensive approach to investigation. With good organisation and facilities, and with the cooperation of you, the patient, the profile can usually be completed within a couple of months. After completion, it is hoped that appropriate therapy can be suggested, discussed, agreed and organised.

Subsequent consultations

How subsequent consultations are conducted and when and what happens will depend on what is to take place. If you are to have tests performed, you should be provided with written and verbal briefing about each at your previous visit. Each follow-up visit is likely also to include discussion of the implications of the latest results and where you could to go next, if at all.

When all your investigations have been completed, and during and after therapy (if any), review appointments (minimum every three months, maximum every six) should be made available for as long as you wish, unless you wish to discontinue or a pregnancy has occurred. Statistics show that the majority of couples conceive fairly quickly and your chances diminish as time progresses. It has been noted that after two years' clinic attendance or four years of trying, IVF excluded, few conceive. One can never say never, but expert help should be on hand to counsel-out if it is deemed to be more in your interests to stop than to continue.

You should also be helped to seek a further opinion elsewhere if you so wish, particularly where facilities have been limited.

Personal Comment

I fully realise and, indeed, empathise with you, that many of you will find investigations time consuming and stressful. However, they must be thorough to be effective. It is important for the infertility team as well as yourselves to acknowledge that tests can sometimes be unpleasant, inconclusive and repetitive. Answers are not always clear-cut, and responses to therapy may be unpredictable and disappointing. No guarantees can be given. It is sad that, even with today's advances, one in twenty of you will be consigned to that meaningless, non-diagnosis of 'unexplained infertility', where empirical treatment and placebo-effect success abound. There can be temptation on all sides to cut corners as time goes on. This is not wise. Forging a verbal contract at the start with your doctor for an agreed, planned approach and sticking to it is in everyone's best interests and will optimise results. I also feel strongly that if, despite the best intentions on all sides, conflict and dissatisfaction set in, it is better for patients to seek early help elsewhere rather than work with a doctor-patient relationship that is likely destined to end in acrimonious tears! You should note, however, that early drop-outs are known to have poorer chances of conceiving.

Chapter 7

Male subfertility

MYTH

The problem is seldom if ever found in the man so why does he need to be involved?

This chapter is concerned with poor semen quality as a potential cause of male-factor infertility. I discuss male sexual dysfunction and physical coital problems in detail in chapter 10 (pages 149-58) and the indications for and use of Donor Insemination(AID) in chapter 11 (pages 195-201).

Incidence

The days have gone when infertility was considered to be a solely female problem. In at least 30% of infertile couples being investigated in a general infertility clinic the male partner has a potentially contributory problem. This can rise to as high as 60% in couples being investigated and treated in tertiary-care clinics where assisted reproduction techniques (ART, see chapter 11, pages 194-246) are practised. Infertility treatment is therefore today focused on both partners together, with male 'gonadal function' (the ability to produce semen of sufficient quality to allow conception) being a key element in this.

Semen production and its control

To understand the options for treating male-factor infertility (sperm problems) it is important for you to have a basic knowledge of normal male genital tract function, how semen is formed and its control.

By birth the testes should have descended into the scrotum (see Figure 4, overleaf) but it is only from puberty onwards, usually around the age of 13-14 (spermarche) that sperm (more correctly, 'spermatozoa' or 'the male gametes') start to be produced conveyor-belt fashion in the testes from the part of it called the 'seminiferous tubule'.

The tubules contain 'spermatogonia', which are the stem cells for sperm-generation. It takes 72 days for spermatozoa to develop fully, from initial primary 'spermatocyte' stages attached to 'Sertoli' cells (specialised 'nurse' cells, also found in the seminiferous tubules), through various 'spermatid' stages to become mature sperm.

Also found in the testes and of vital importance are the Leydig cells. These secrete testosterone. As with ovarian hormone production in women (see chapter 9 and Figure 12, page 121) but, much less fluctuating and not so cyclical in nature, testosterone production is under negative feedback control from the sex hormone luteinising hormone (LH) stimulated and produced in the hypothalamic-pituitary axis in the brain. As the level of testosterone goes up it switches off the production of the pituitary hormone, LH. Then as the level of testosterone falls, more LH is then produced, stimulating more testosterone production.

Spermatogenesis and Sertoli cell function are principally controlled by a different hormone – 'follicle stimulating' hormone (FSH). This is also produced by the pituitary gland, again subject to a feedback switch-off-on hormonal mechanism, this time called 'inhibin'. Some interaction between FSH and LH is also suspected at the target organ level.

The sperm leave the testes via the 'epididymal ducts' and approximately 10-14 days after this enter the 'vas deferens'. This is the tube taking the sperm from epididymis to penis. The majority of sperm are stored here pre-ejaculation.

While sperm are produced in the testes, at ejaculation only 5-7% of the

Figure 4 Diagram of male genital tract

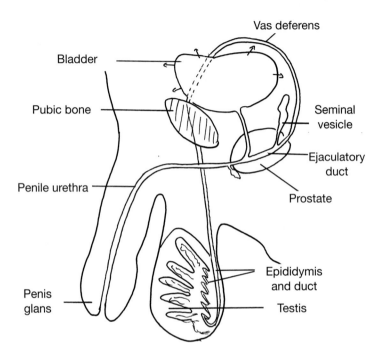

seminal fluid (semen) actually consists of sperm. The rest of the semen is made up of secretions from other organs containing vital substances for the sperm's final maturation, motility and fertilisation capability (known as 'capacitation'). The main contributors to semen are other organs that are passed on the way to the ejaculatory ducts and penile 'urethra', especially the prostate (10-30%) and seminal vesicles (40-60%).

The final semen composition comes into being only as ejaculation occurs. It is initially coagulated (clotted) so that it is retained in the female vagina after deposition rather than it running straight out again and being wasted.This enhances the chance of pregnancy. Liquefaction occurs some 30 minutes later.

The necessary male sexual response, ejaculation and emission and related problems and their management are discussed fully in chapter 10 (pages 147-58). However, in the context of this chapter it is sufficient to say that they are under the control of the central nervous system and locally through a complex reflex nerve arc. The nerves come out from the spine in two places, firstly just above the top of the pelvis (known as levels T (thorax) 12 - L (lumbar) 3) and secondly from the sides at the lowest part of the back (the sacrum at levels S2 — S4). These nerves, plus an intact blood supply to the area, are essential to the process of successful penile erection and ejaculation.

Words used to describe types of abnormal semen quality

'Azoospermia' is the term used when no sperm are found, 'oligo-zoospermia' when numbers are lower than normal, 'asthenozoosper-mia' if motility (ability to move) is poor and 'necrospermia' if all appear dead. 'Polyspermia' is used when density is very high (more than 150 million per millilitre).

The causes behind such abnormalities in semen may be categorised in a number of different ways. Whatever system is used, (for simplicity, in this book the various organs of the male reproductive anatomy (Figure 4) are the reference points), the categories are not mutually exclusive.

Causes of abnormal semen quality

In the majority of men (said to be some 65%), the cause of testicular malfunction is unknown or cannot be detected.

Testicular causes of semen abnormalities

Absence
Absence of both testes is rare, other than following 'orchidectomy' (removal) for cancer, torsion (twisting) complications, or trauma. Absence

or loss of one testis should not affect the quality of semen being produced provided that the other is functioning normally.

Malposition (undescended testes)

The testes function best at a temperature below core body temperature (that is, at 35°C). Therefore, if they have failed to descend along the correct pathway fully by birth into the scrotum and are retained within the body, (this is called cryptorchidism) by the time puberty is reached, their ability to produce sperm may have been destroyed by being in the overheated (for them) normal body temperature environment (37°C). This is the commonest and most easily deduced cause of primary testicular disease. Unless this problem is addressed early in life, irreversible damage may result, with complete loss of sperm-producing cells leading to azoospermia and also an increased risk of testicular cancer.

Totally undescended, or partially descended, testes may be unilateral (on one side) or bilateral (on both sides). They are responsible for some 20% of cases of male-factor infertility. Early detection is essential if infertility is to be prevented. Whoever does the first post-birth examination should be on the lookout for it and a parent can check at bath time during the first few months of life.

The differential diagnosis of ectopic testis, where the testis ends outside the scrotum after a normal initial descent, is much rarer.

Infectious diseases

Any severe illness may influence semen quality temporarily via a general effect on body function. The testis is, however, not immune from infections acting specifically on the organ itself. Acute infective inflammatory illnesses of the testes are given the name 'orchitis'. When they occur, they can destroy or obstruct internal testicular function. This includes infections such as mumps. However, only some 12% of males who get mumps-orchitis affecting both testes will be rendered infertile. Tuberculosis and leprosy may damage any organ in the body directly, including the testes or, in the latter case by setting up an auto-immune reaction producing antibodies to the sperm.

Physical damage
Trauma

Severe trauma to the testes and their blood supply may lead to direct failure of function. Removal can become necessary. Sometimes this is also needed when the testis becomes spontaneously twisted (torsion). In this very painful condition (where the pain may be referred to the abdomen rather than be local), if the testis is not untwisted quickly the blood supply can become cut off to the affected testis, which can then become gangrenous, necessitating removal.

Cancer

Apart from direct testicular damage due to cancer itself, some types of chemotherapy and radiotherapy from childhood onwards are also highly likely to cause physical damage to testicular germ cells and their sperm production function. This may lead to azoospermia. The types of cancer whose treatment leads to this situation are mostly testicular tumours, lymphomas, leukaemias, and any where bone marrow transplantation is contemplated.

The damage may become permanent in the case of direct radiation to the area. With the commonly used chemotherapeutic agents, especially the family of drugs known as the 'alkylating agents', it may also be permanent or temporary; whichever, return to normal quality is unpredictable in terms of time scale. For this reason it is now suggested that all those who find themselves in such circumstances should enquire about semen banking in advance of cancer treatment to attempt to preserve ability to have children in the future (see chapter 11, pages 203, 208, 231).

Hormone deficiencies

As I said at the start of this chapter, spermatogenesis and its associated hormonal secretions are under the control of the follicle stimulating hormone (FSH) and luteinising hormone (LH), both produced by the pituitary gland in the brain under hypothalamic-pituitary axis control (see Figure 12, page 121). Abnormalities or failure in the output of hormones from the axis glands due to congenital defects, infection, trauma or tumour formation in the area may therefore affect spermatogenesis and testosterone production.

FSH and LH production may be poor from the start of life, be stopped directly or when vital cells in the hypothalamic-pituitary-axis are destroyed through pressure from a tumour sited nearby, for example, or a failure in blood supply ('hypogonadotrophic hypogonadism'). Conversely, gonadotrophic production will go up if the target organ, the testis itself, fails (akin to what happens in the female at the menopause). However, this has to be differentiated from where there is a tumour in the pituitary that secretes excess FSH.

The pituitary also secretes other hormones that control other systems in the body including growth, the thyroid and the adrenal glands. Excessive secretion of some of these hormones can sometimes also affect control of sperm production. These include particularly growth hormone and a hormone called the adrenocorticotrophic hormone (ACTH) that stimulates the hormones of the adrenal glands (cortisol especially).

On the male hormone testosterone secretion side, with conditions such as testosterone-secreting tumours of the testes and adrenal glands, the excess testosterone will cause a virtually permanent down-regulation situation and therefore the pituitary sex hormone function (principally LH but possibly also FSH) is switched off. This may also happen with renal dialysis, and with anabolic steroid abuse, as seen sometimes in athletes and body builders. It can also happen with liver disease, which can result in failure to handle and detoxify sex hormones normally and thus affect FSH and LH production.

Occupational and environmental causes

Solid evidence has now accumulated to relate certain occupations to male-factor infertility – for example, work involving contact with radiation. Exposure to over 100 rads will lead to 90% of men getting azoospermia. Effects are similar with exposure to agricultural or industrial toxins (e.g. DBCP, EDB, DDT and lead; the latter can occur with people making car batteries, for example). Awareness has led to some substances such as DDT being withdrawn from the market. In many countries, but unfortunately not all, health and safety regulations have set down what precautions should be taken and the amount of allowable exposure as toxicity is usually dose and time related.

In addition, it has been suggested recently that semen quality in men is generally deteriorating, possibly as a result of ingesting an excess of the female hormone oestrogen, added deliberately or via inadvertent contamination within the food chain to meat and fish. Extensive research is ongoing and there appears to be some truth in this, but do not stop eating meat and fish yet as comparisons of present-day sperm counts with those of yesteryear are problematic. Few large population studies of sperm counts from years ago are available for comparison and, as discussed later in this chapter, methodology has changed somewhat.

Smoking and street drugs

Tobacco smoking, marijuana, cocaine, heroin and methadone have all been found to be associated with lower than normal sperm counts. What is damaged is unclear in all these situations; the effect may be direct on the testis cells or, in the case of marijuana, associated with low testosterone levels.

With smoking, nicotine is implicated, but the situation is often multifactorial and the available data do not conclusively show that male fertility is decreased. A dose-dependent reduction of 22% in semen quality compared to non-smokers has, however, been measured and in another study at a general infertility clinic, 41% of male partner attendees who smoked had reduced sperm count densities compared with 26% of non-smokers.

Genetic abnormalities affecting sperm production

Genetic causes due to chromosomal abnormalities (see chapter 2) are present from birth but may come to light only when a man is investigated for infertility. The commonest found are Kleinefelter's syndrome (3-4% of all azoospermic men) and Noonan's syndrome. Kleinefelter's syndrome is where the man is discovered to have an extra female X chromosome (XXY instead of XY), and Noonan's syndrome is where the man is found to have no male Y chromosome (XO instead of XY).

Other chromosomal abnormalities such as XYY and XX males are more in focus today, and others are coming to light as a result of improvements in method and availability of genetic testing (see later on in this chapter). Their discovery is also driven by the need to investigate before resorting to ICSI (intra-cytoplasmic sperm injection) with male-factor infertility. The principal abnormalities are translocations (in 5% of oligospermic men, where one or more of the chromosomes moves from one site to another) and Y chromosome deletions (absences of genes somewhere along the normal Y male chromosome structure). Chromosomal abnormalities have been found in 7.3% of men with azoospermia and, in my practice, overall with sperm counts of up to five million, in 3.5% with 40% translocations (see pages 184, 215).

Thought to be genetically based, and linked to men also suffering from sinus, respiratory tract and heart diseases, is Kartagener's syndrome. In this situation rather than azoospermia or oligozoospermia, the sperm numbers appear normal but are immotile (cannot move) due to lack of normal tail function.

Obstruction of the outflow ducts from testis to penis

Problems with the outflow ducts are a common cause of male-factor infertility. They account for some 15% of cases. Intra-testicular (inside the testes) causes are rare (2%). The most common obstruction sites are the epididymis and the vas deferens (see Figure 4). If this occurs on both sides (bilateral) and is complete this will lead to what is called 'obstructive azoospermia'. In this situation, spermatogenesis is usually still going on in the testis itself behind the blockage but the sperm cannot get out. However, through the development of ICSI (see chapter 11, page 210) sperm are potentially extractible directly from the testis or the vas and can be used for attempts at conception.

Congenital absence or obstruction of the ducts

The epididymis may be congenitally absent but more commonly the problem is congenital absence of the two vas deferens. This accounts for 10% of all causes of obstructive azoospermia. This is a very common finding in men with the genetic disease cystic fibrosis. In addition to all the lung, gall bladder and pancreatic problems that such sufferers get due to excessively viscid (thick) mucus secretions, in males, if there is also bilateral absence of the vas, semen analysis will show azoospermia, although the underlying testes are usually functioning normally.

Other underlying hereditary but thankfully rare obstructive duct syndromes can sometimes, often in an unknown way, link problems in different body system. The commonest is Young's syndrome, a combination of azoospermia due to epididymis obstruction, obstructive sinusitis and obstructive lung disease that leads to chronic respiratory infection and lung tissue destruction (bronchiectasis).

Infection

Acute infection, from many different viruses, bacteria and unicellular organisms, can cause obstructive blockage. These include those transmitted sexually, such as *Gonococcus* and *Chlamydia trachomatis*. The word 'itis' which indicates inflammation is attached to the infection site such as in 'epididymitis'. If blockage occurs it may remain long after the infection has gone.

Chronic disease such as tuberculosis (TB) and sarcoidosis may affect the epididymis as well as the vas and seminal vesicles. The organs then feel thicker. Azoospermia is the result. Sperm production itself may also be affected .

Trauma

Injuries in the scrotal area may cause epididymal obstruction directly or due to pressure from a clot that may form after bleeding. More commonly, the site is in the vas and 'iatrogenic' (caused by medical or surgical intervention), such as a vasectomy or inadvertent damage to the vas while attempting to operate on a child to correct undescended testes.

Retrograde ejaculation

Retrograde ejaculation occurs when most or all of the seminal ejaculate goes into the bladder rather than out through the tip of the penile urethra. It therefore presents at first on a routine semen analysis attempt as azoospermia and it therefore appropriate, and convenient, to consider it here.

The cause is often unknown. At ejaculation, the bladder neck normally closes. This stops semen from entering the bladder. Consequently, if the bladder neck is traumatically damaged or not working for some other reason, such as damage to the sympathetic nervous system as a result of pelvic surgery, diabetes or spinal injury, it becomes 'incompetent' (no longer closes properly). Backward seminal flow at ejaculation can also occur following operations on the prostate, especially near the bladder neck, which can be damaged. In this situation, a masturbatory semen sample volume will be lower than normal, with at the most only a few dead sperm found after a search. However, finding live sperm in a post-coital urine sample is diagnostic and treatment may then become a possibility (see Optimal use of available semen, page 58, and chapter 11, page 202).

Varicocele

A varicocele is a collection of varicose veins, usually found on the left side of the testis. It is formed from the veins that drain the area and is very common in the normal population (some 10%) but found more often (up to 35%) in men with poor quality semen. Testicular size and volume can be found to be reduced where there is a varicocele, but semen only sometimes appears to be affected: sometimes the quality is reduced compared with that of men without varicoceles, but it may still be within the present parameters of 'normality'. It is fair to say its place as a cause of male-factor infertility has still not been fully determined.

Diagnosis

General

The usual way of dealing with any medical problem (see chapter 5) is for the doctor to start by taking the patient's 'history', moving on to physical examination. The combination of these two may point to appropriate tests that will help with diagnosis. Treatment then follows, if available, desirable and desired. I follow this order in chapters 8-10 and also here, in chapter 7, although the sequence is sometimes not what happens in an infertile man despite it now being acknowledged that infertility is a couple's problem. Although the situation is improving, this is because in many cases the female partner will still be the one to have made the approach for help. Semen analysis is then ordered immediately, male unseen, after her first consultation. In these circumstances, unless he already realises from a past history of illness that there could be a problem and consults a doctor himself initially, it can come as a bewildering and unpleasant surprise for the man to be summoned to the infertility clinic to discuss a potential problem of which he was hitherto been oblivious. The first stage in finding problems in the male is often therefore an investigation (semen analysis) rather than the classical history-taking and physical examination.

History

In some instances, it may be a urologist with a male fertility interest who takes matters further, for others it can be a gynaecologist with 'andrological' (male infertility) training. Whichever, this is likely to be in a tertiary care centre. Sometimes both will get involved on different aspects of the problem.

The clue to what the problem is and to its underlying cause may emerge from answers to specific questions that relate to the causes of male factor infertility discussed above. These include past operations in the area, especially inguinal hernia repair as a child, radiotherapy or chemotherapy, medications, infections or general diseases such as diabetes and TB. A sexual history will also be taken as it may also be revealing (see chapter 10, page 151), as may the man's occupation, lifestyle and a family history of male problems with conception.

Physical examination

In all initial fertility consultations but especially where male subfertility is suspected, the doctor will note if clothing may be causing a problem by being too restricting on the gonads. Excess height and a high arched palate can be associated with the genetic condition Marfan's syndrome and growth hormone excess can lead to acromegaly, both of which are associated with defective sperm production.

The potentially infertile male can expect to have a full examination of all body systems – cardiac, respiratory, nervous, plus chest and abdomen in all situations where the semen analysis is found to be abnormal. This is to assess general health and wellbeing as well as possibly identify underlying general and local disease that may be relevant. It may include a rectal examination in order to 'palpate' (feel) some of the genital tract organs, such as the prostate.

The genital area is, however, the main focus of attention. You will be asked to stand upright with no clothes covering this region. The doctor will look for anatomical abnormalities such as apparent absence of testes, small testicular volume or a penile deformity, such as 'hypospadias' (where the urine and therefore semen outlet is not at the tip of the penis). S/he will also look to see if there is a varicocele in the scrotum (the skin covered sac containing the testes and epididymis) and attempt to palpate the vas.

This history and physical examination may indicate what further in-depth investigations are needed, including possibly more semen analyses.

Chapter 7

Investigations

Semen analysis
Semen analysis (alias the 'spermiogram') is the cornerstone of male fertility investigations. Anxious couples may find home kits can be useful as an initial pre-GP basic screening test to see if sperm are there or not. Results must, however, be interpreted with caution.

The true, gold-standard, diagnostically reliable test of male function is a full formal semen analysis. This can be performed only in a laboratory with appropriate expertise on a semen sample produced by masturbation into a sterile sterylene (plastic) container. This sample should be produced up to three hours before analysis and at an interval of two to three days after the last ejaculation (reckoned to be best recovery time to maximise semen quality). You can reasonably expect to be given written instructions and an appropriate container by your clinic. Results should be out by the following day.

The test has been refined over the years to include sperm antibody evaluation and the detection of infection in the seminal fluid, but the main criteria ('parameters') continue to be measures of sperm 'quality'. It is important to be aware that following scientific review, levels now said to be 'normal' are lower than the normal values quoted in the past.

These 'normal' values are relative; most of the parameters measured depend on an observer. Each laboratory should have its own reference range for the population it serves. Most importantly, abnormalities when found do not automatically condemn the male to having no chance of ever fathering a child. Female fertility potential also comes into the equation.

The presently quoted 'normal' main values are, as stated by the World Health Organisation (WHO) in 1999: a volume of 2.0 millilitres (ml) or more; a density count (number per ml) concentration of over twenty million (20,000,000); with a total count of over forty million (40,000,000), of which at least 50% are motile or 25% are moving forward (progressive motility) and 15% or more appear of normal morphology (shape) and 75% are alive.

49

These WHO parameters include the controversial subject of 'anti-sperm antibodies' (see Chapter 10, the cervical factor, pages 136-44). The 'mixed antiglobulin reaction' (MAR) is the basic test for this problem and thought to be positive when added particles stick (cause clotting) to more than over 80% of sperm (normally fewer than 50%). This can be followed up by the 'immunobead' test, which is more specific in terms of type of antibody present (normally fewer than 50% with beads bound).

Sending samples to the lab to look for bacterial infection in the semen is justified only if the man's history suggests infection may be present, or if a high number of white cells (WHO states over one million per ml) are seen in the semen-analysis sample. Over 90% of semen will contain infective organisms. This is usually due to skin contamination from masturbatory friction at production, although infection in the prostate gland can possibly also be a cause.

Problems with semen analysis as a specific test for male infertility
Despite being the gold-standard cornerstone test for male infertility, semen analysis is not always reliable or reproducible. There can be wide inter-observer differences. In fact, it illustrates very well two of the big gaps we have in infertility investigations – namely, what is a 'normal sperm' and when is a male truly infertile if sperm are being produced at all no matter how few? Steps can be taken to minimise this situation however. A minimum of two semen specimens is needed for any judgement to be made. If any of the basic parameters still fall below 'normality' after these analyses, further discussion and investigation are needed for individuals who wish to go on.

Semen analysis may also not be diagnostic if carried out by a laboratory that does not have the appropriate level of expertise, for example, to investigate the seminal plasma fully. It may be worth reassuring yourself about the level of specialist expertise of the laboratory used and if they use external quality-control.

The most common and easily avoidable problem with semen analysis is the sample being unrepresentative. This can occur because of insufficient time having been left from the last ejaculation (2–3 days to maximise semen recovery) or because of spillage on production, and may be compounded by the lack of suitable discrete facilities for production in a clinic. This is the preferred place (as far at the health professionals are concerned) for specimen production as the semen can then be easily and quickly stored at a suitable temperature and for the correct length of time before being analysed. Clear instructions beforehand should minimise the chances of spillage, but home may be preferable for individuals affected by the pressure of producing a sample in the clinic as long as the sample is kept warm until reaching the laboratory.

Diagnosing possible male factors without masturbatory sample production

Alternatives to semen specimen production by masturbation in the clinic, or at home, may need to be considered as a last resort if failure to produce by this method persists or there is a religious barrier to it. These include obtaining and examining a post-coital condom specimen. For this a non-lubricated, non-spermicidal condom should be used as the spermicide that is present in normal condoms will kill the sperm and thus give a false motility result.

The other alternative is to perform a post-coital test (see chapter 10, pages 137-8). If the post-coital test is positive (multiple motile progressing sperms seen in ovulatory type cervical mucus), and couples are shown this on the spot under the microscope, the result can also be valuable psychologically. It will demonstrate to a couple that sperm are being produced, that they have been deposited in the vagina and have reached the cervix and thus are at least capable of potentially entering the uterus alive.

The data obtained will not be so accurate and not so many parameters can be tested as in a formal semen analysis. But, where it is possible to do both, results obtained will correlate with those from semen analysis in terms of count and motility estimations in over 90% of cases. When it does not, this is a signal to check the semen again whatever past results.

Blood tests
Hormones

Hormonal investigations may point to a cause and determine what, if any, treatment can be offered. This is especially in men with azoospermia. A basic profile of FSH and LH plus testosterone can be quite expensive and may need to be repeated. It may show that the fault lies in the brain (low levels of FSH and/or LH), which is potentially treatable, or with testicular failure (high FSH and/or LH) which is likely not. If hormone levels are found to be normal, this suggests spermatogenesis is going on even if repeated semen samples show azoospermia. Other reasons such as a duct blockage will then need to be sought.

Chromosome tests

Blood is usually only taken in infertility situations when an underlying genetic reason for subfertility is suspected. Indeed, despite the expense, chromosome analysis is now considered a diagnostic essential in men with absent or very low sperm counts, especially those who wish to use ICSI (intra-cytoplasmic sperm injection) to try to procreate. If found positive, genetic counselling will then be needed so there is clarity as to the potential risk that is being taken of transmitting the fault to an offspring. (See also chapter 11, page 215.)

Epididymal aspiration/testicular biopsy

Epididymal aspiration and testicular biopsy were popular diagnostic tools years ago.They then became unfashionable as hormone tests were able to supply most of the information needed to determine the cause of semen problems or the possible presence of hidden spermatogenesis in men with azoospermia. However, in light of modern ART treatments and particularly ICSI (see chapter 11, pages 211-12), these tests have come back into vogue as part of potential therapy.

Both approaches are usually performed under local anaesthetic or sedo-analgesia (see chapter 11, page 219). Epididymal aspiration is relevant if there is a blockage in the vas and palpation suggests an accumulated pocket of sperm is present. Testicular biopsy is the ultimate determinant of fertility potential and is used for all other potential blockage situations or if testicular size or hormone assays suggest testicular failure is not complete. Multiple biopsies may, however, be needed and the danger is that the only bit of functioning testicular tissue may be removed forever. The aim is to show whether there is any sperm production capable of being utilised towards an attempt at conception (see pages 207, 212, 229).

Although testicular biopsy can be of diagnostic value, with possible future rather than current treatment in mind, it is best carried out in a clinic with sperm cryo-preservation on site so that if sperm are found, they can immediately be cryo-preserved for a later attempt at conception. Once biopsy has been carried out, three to six months should elapse to get over testicular shock before an extraction is again attempted.

Treatment options

Where no treatment is possible

Where organs are absent or there is significant destruction of testicular tissues, there is no treatment that will improve sperm production. For male hypogonadism (testosterone deficiency) itself, testosterone analogues (artificial equivalents) are available to treat the symptoms of male hormone deficiency but these will not help sperm production. Even if therapy is possible, it may not be advisable or acceptable if, for example, there is a high risk of passing on a serious hereditary genetic disease to any offspring.

In all these cases the alternatives of no treatment, adoption and donor insemination (see pages 196, 253) need to be discussed. Expert genetic and infertility counselling may be helpful and can be very important, as in all situations where 'no further treatment' is advised.

Malpositioned or undescended testes

A testis can remain malpositioned from very early in development. It can be ectopic, where an abnormal route is taken and surgical removal may be necessary, especially if trauma occurs.

More commonly one or both testes may be maldescended and not enter the scrotum at all. They may remain anywhere along the line of descent from high in the abdomen where they are first formed (the genital ridge) to the entrance to the scrotum if descent has not been completed during the baby's life in his mother's uterus birth (cryptorchidism).

If the testes are found (as is commonest) near to the scrotum, in an area between the top of the leg and the abdomen called the inguinal ring region, it maybe possible to operate and bring them into the scrotal sac. This operation is called orchidopexy.

However, it is now felt important for parents to realise that this operation needs to be performed pre-puberty if there is to be any real chance of good spermatogenesis in the future. Indeed, the fashion now is if possible to perform this between 18 and 24 months of age as this seems to be more effective in maintaining future function and in preventing the onset later of testicular tumours.

If it is not possible to perform orchidopexy, and perhaps more germane to the infertile male reading this chapter, the concensus is that considering removal of the testis may be better at this stage of life, especially if it is unilateral or sited in the abdomen when some 30% may become malignant. However, if both testes are removed, androgen replacement therapy may become necessary. After puberty orchidopexy is not warranted as it is by then too late to preserve testicular function.

Where treatment is possible

Historically, where treatment was considered possible, the options were divided into those that aimed to improve the quality of the sperm and hence the chances of natural conception and those directed towards seeing what could be done using the sperm already available.

Attempting to improve quality of sperm production

Before the advent of IVF and especially ICSI (see chapter 11, pages 211-13), attempting to improve the quality of sperm used to be the approach of choice. Results were poor, with a success rate (that is, conception achieved) of only 10%. However, there are some proven useful treatments in some situations that should not be ignored in their own right. Indeed, some (the latest are anti-oxidants) remain also as a positive adjunct to present-day assisted reproductive techniques (ART).

General measures

In addition to dealing with any general diseases found, your doctor should still attend to indicators of general body and mind wellbeing such as weight and diet and will advise on the avoidance of clothing that restricts the testes. Stopping the use of recreational drugs, especially cannabis, and of anabolic steroids is essential. Any such substances can lower sperm counts to zero during intake. The effects can persist for some considerable time after intake has stopped.

Surgery

Ligation (tieing off) of a varicocele may still have a part to play. The former is at present time thought to be indicated only for a large varicocele that is uncomfortable. Ultrasound may help make the decision as to whether to operate or not. The incision can be either in the scrotum or more commonly above it.

Operations on duct obstructions such as the epididymis can be useful and still should be considered pre ICSI. This is particularly pertinent where the outflow tract is obstructed in the vas deferens region due to infection or where there has been previous surgery, especially vasectomy.

Where a vasectomy is the cause of azoospermia and reversal is possible, this should always be the first choice approach, although the likelihood of success declines if it is over two years since the vasectomy was originally done.

'Vasovasostomy', which is where the obstruction in the vas is cut out and the two open tube ends stitched together again microsurgically, could be also of benefit after an infection if testicular function is normal.

Antibiotic therapy for semen infections

In the past antibiotic treatment was claimed to improve sperm motility. Nowadays, only culture counts over 10,000 or white cell counts over 1,000,000/ml are considered positive indicators that the man needs antibiotic therapy. As with most genital tract infections, the source (nidus) where the infective organisms are sited is likely to be in an organ such as the prostate.

Lipid-soluble tetracyclines such as the doxycycline family are favoured unless the individual concerned is known to be allergic to these. They counteract most of the usual common infective organisms found and reach the site best.

Hormone therapy

Hormone therapy is the treatment of choice where low levels of FSH and LH indicate very low pituitary activity affecting testicular sperm production. Replacement of the deficiency aimed at restarting sperm production where these pituitary gonadotrophic hormones are absent, or supplementing them when very low, can be attempted using long-term injectable gonadotrophins. These contain FSH with or without LH or human gonadotrophic hormone (hCG). The effect can sometimes be good but only where the problem is 'hypogonadotrophic hypogonadism' (under-production of gonadotrophin by the pituitary gland; see page 60).

However, stimulation of the testes with other fertility drugs does not seem to work, unlike the good results seen with fertility drugs such as clomiphene citrate in women (chapter 9). Other substances such as male testosterone derivatives (androgenic hormonal supplements), vitamins and minerals such as zinc (chapter 12), or steroids (as used in the presence of 'anti-sperm antibodies', see chapter 10, page 142), have never been shown to be more effective than placebo or no treatment.

Optimal use of available semen
Artificial insemination (AI)

In the past, AI was a favoured method used in men with oligo-zoospermia (lower than normal sperm count). Semen was deposited into the cervix, or, after washing most of the seminal fluid off first, sperm were deposited into the uterus (IUI) (see chapter 11, page 202 and Figures 13-14, pages 200 and 202). It gave poor results and has been superseded by ICSI (see chapter 11, pages 202, 211-13).

Before IVF became available, attempts were made to improve AI results in men with oligo- or asthenozoospermia, by accumulating and cryo-preserving a number of semen samples. When sufficient quantities had been obtained, samples were pooled together, the aim being to use these all together for AI at an appropriate time in the cycle.

Such desperate measures seldom if every truly worked, and this was also the case with attempts at enhancing semen quality pre AI with additives such as caffeine, even though adding these directly to the semen sample improved motility considerably, but temporarily; most sperm did not then live beyond a further 20 minutes.

Where circulating sperm antibodies were found, couples used to be advised to use condom coitus for a few months to allow the antibody levels to regress without semen contact, or by washing the sample first if sperm-antibodies were present. Not only have the tests then used on the female to detect the 'sperm-antibodies' been debunked, and superseded by direct semen tests, but results were awful (see pages 141-2).

AI has, however, remained on the list of current legitimate available treatments, albeit for use in different circumstances than previously. AI, or ICSI, is used when semen has been cryo-banked (put into cold-storage at -196°C) before cancer therapy and later on the patient wants to conceive (only some 30% of men actually return to try). It is also used for a few cycles (mandatory in some clinics) before embarking on IVF, but only where the sperm count is normal, and especially where there is 'unexplained infertility' (see chapter 11, page 206).

AI is also appropriate for retrograde ejaculation if drugs that aim to stimulate the possibly malfunctioning nervous control of the bladder neck (sympathomimetic types of the pseudoephidrine class) do not reverse the problem. Urine alkalysing agents are taken first (generally potassium citrate) as the normal acidity of urine would kill the sperm. The bladder has to be emptied before and after coitus or masturbation to climax. The second urine sample, containing the ejaculated sperm, can then be used by the couple in the privacy of their home for DIY AI (see chapter 11, pages 198, 203).

IVF/ICSI

IVF/ICSI is described in greater detail in chapter 11 (see pages 209-46). While general thinking on male-factor infertility was transformed by the advent of IVF in 1978, results continued to be disappointing in men with oligozoospermia and significantly lower than for other indications for IVF such as tubal blockage. Matters altered significantly in 1992, when the direct injection of a single sperm into a single egg (ICSI) was first reported. This technique has supplanted almost all other therapies for male factor infertility and can now give procreative hope in some situations where in the past it might have seemed impossible.

Prognosis for male factor infertility therapies

General issues

As I said at the beginning of the book (chapter 3), in attempting to give an idea of the chances of achieving pregnancy and avoiding complications there are a great many factors that can influence success, including especially the partner's contribution. In looking at the chances of success, I have, for simplicity's sake, assumed that the female partner has no problems (chapters 8-10) and that treatments are carried out fully and properly. However, even if the female partner's contribution is left out of the equation the true efficacy of any specific therapy for many infertile men remains impossible to quantify. There are the confounding variables of general health and age in either partner, length of their infertility and past reproductive history potentially to be considered.

As in all therapeutic situations, before starting on the journey, it is also worth checking whether any treatment that has been suggested to you is backed by positive results from a 'blinded, placebo-controlled' scientific trial (grade A). This is the only true scientific validation of therapy but it may be impossible always to find. Few such studies, have been carried out in any branch of infertility, never mind the male. Lesser evidence, such as is provided by other good observational studies (grade B), or more limited expert opinion shared by respected authorities (grade C), may have to be accepted instead. You can of course decide not to embark on treatment at all.

Where no treatment is possible

Sometimes active therapy cannot be provided or it fails and nothing else can be suggested. As is natural, signs associated with stress and depression, (see chapter 10, page 164) may set in. Taking stock with your partner over time rather than instantly will pay dividends as will the help of counsellors trained specifically in the area and in looking at alternatives.

Attempting to improve quality of semen production

General measures

Whether active treatment to improve semen quality can be offered or not, general measures may help. These include improving lifestyle, and eliminating toxins and chemical agents known to be detrimental including recreational drugs and tobacco. As I have already said, the evidence concerning recreational drugs is strong; for tobacco smoking quantification is more difficult. Although improvement in semen quality is generally asserted in most papers on the subject, many of these are concerned with optimising production that was already within normal parameters.

Surgery

The data on undescended testes is clear and devastatingly negative in terms of sperm production potential unless orchidopexy operation (testes tied down in scrotum) is possible and carried out at a very young age, when the prognosis for some future spermatogenesis can be excellent.

Up-to-date figures that quantify the results of other different surgical treatments are, however, difficult to find even locally and international success rates based on sufficient numbers of cases are virtually non-existent. However, operations to clear obstruction of the outflow ducts (vas deferens etc), such as microsurgical vasovasostomy, do give results on a par with individuals who have no blockage (that is normal fecundity), but not where the blockage is as a result of chronic infection.

Reversal of vasectomy can be equally successful if the blood supply is good. However, if sperm antibodies have developed over time, the chances of pregnancy seem to get smaller.

As I have said earlier, surgery for a varicocele should be considered only if the varicocele is very large and causing discomfort. Semen quality may improve after the procedure.

Hormone treatment to improve semen quality

Only one of the hormonal treatments currently on offer has been scientifically shown to come up to or exceed the expected placebo effect, or the use of ICSI, in improving sperm quality. This is gonadotrophin therapy, but only for hypogonadotrophic hypogonadism (under-production of gonadotrophin by the pituitary gland). This has been scientifically shown to come up to or to sometimes exceed the overall expected placebo effect of up to perhaps 30% (see chapter 5, page 26) in stimulating semen production and achieving pregnancy.

Optimal use of available sperm (AIH and ICSI)

Even using normal sperm and IUI with or without ovulation stimulation, 15% is still the universally accepted figure for AIH pregnancies being achieved. Where sperm quality is poor this success rate is significantly lower (chapter 11, page 207). Using frozen semen does seem to lower the chances with AI but not with ICSI. For ICSI for a male-factor problem, it is reasonable to expect complication rates and prognosis similar to or better than the overall mean multi-national results (European Society of Human Reproduction and Embryology (ESHRE)) for all ICSI of some 29.8% of cycles transferred resulting in pregnancy (depending on the age of the female partner; see chapter 11, page 242).

Personal Comment

In my view a semen test should be carried out at the earliest opportunity to determine, or rule out, a male-factor cause of infertility before continuing on with investigations in the woman. Refusal by a man to participate is valid grounds for discontinuing investigations altogether. However, male-factor infertility largely remains a mystery with many unknowns deserving exploration. New research aimed at producing better therapies virtually stopped as ICSI came on stream as its results were spectacularly good compared with anything available in the past. However, thorough investigation of cause is still good medical practice and sometimes alternatives can and should be given their chance first. If these cure, every coitus thereafter gives the chance of pregnancy whereas with ICSI this is confined to the fresh treatment cycle with possible backup from stored frozen embryos. There are also still some questions about ICSI in terms of indications for it and the health of the children it produces. Where no treatment can be offered, counselling is absolutely essential to discuss options before discharge from the clinic.

Chapter 8

Utero-tubal factors

MYTH

IVF is always the optimal treatment for all fallopian tube problems.

Introduction

The fallopian tubes and uterus share a common embryological origin and are found together in the abdominal (peritoneal) cavity. They are joined anatomically and as they are usually initially investigated together, it is traditional to describe them and their associated problems together as the 'utero-tubal factor' in infertility. However, in this chapter I shall consider them as distinct organs with separate functions, problems and therapeutic solutions, although this may result in some repetition.

SECTION I: PROBLEMS WITH THE UTERUS

Anatomy

Excluding the neck of the womb, or 'cervix' (2.5 cm in length), which I consider in detail in chapter 10, it is easiest for practical purposes to think of the uterus (see Figure 5 opposite; size 7.5 x 0.5 x 2.5 cm) as consisting of three distinct layers, each with different important functions: the

Figure 5 Diagrams of the female genital tract

Diagram of female reproductive organs

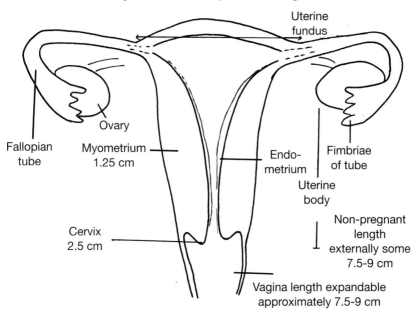

Uterine fundus

Ovary

Fallopian tube

Myometrium 1.25 cm

Endo-metrium

Fimbriae of tube

Uterine body

Non-pregnant length externally some 7.5-9 cm

Cervix 2.5 cm

Vagina length expandable approximately 7.5-9 cm

Lateral cross section of pelvic organs

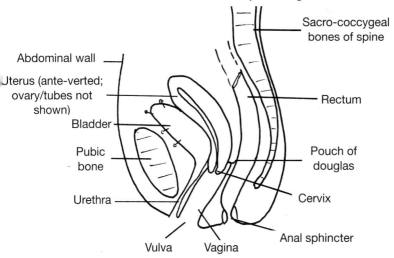

Sacro-coccygeal bones of spine

Abdominal wall

Uterus (ante-verted; ovary/tubes not shown)

Bladder

Rectum

Pubic bone

Pouch of douglas

Urethra

Cervix

Vulva

Vagina

Anal sphincter

peritoneal outer covering, the myometrium (middle muscular layer), and the inner lining – the endometrium. The myometrium is the muscular wall of the uterus and is 1.25 cm thick. The endometrium varies in thickness during the menstrual cycle.

In the majority of women the anterior (front) length of the vagina from its entrance at the vulva is about 7.5 cm up to where the cervix enters near the top. At the back it is some 9 cm in length. This difference allows a pool of semen to collect after intercourse near the cervical entrance to the uterus while the woman is lying down, thus facilitating the passage of sperm upwards in the female genital tract.

The uterus, positioned in the abdomen at the top of the vagina, is in the majority of women tilted forwards ('anteverted'). Equally normally, however, it may tilt backwards ('retroverted'). This is of no consequence unless the backwards tilt is the result of being pulled backwards by a complicating external problem such as endometriosis (see pages 96-104) or adhesions. (Adhesions are bands of tissue that form as part of the body's defence mechanisms in a response to an inflammatory process, forming a wall around the affected area to prevent spread.) There is no evidence to support the corrective surgery ('suspension operations') used in the past to correct an uncomplicated retroversion found in an infertile woman.

Main reasons for reproductive difficulty associated with the uterus

Problems associated with the myometrium

Congenital abnormalities

Congenital abnormalities generally affect the shape of the uterus (see Figure 6, page 66). They are common, affecting 7-8% of women, but are a rare cause of infertility. They are more likely to be implicated in recurrent miscarriage (see chapter 10, pages 182-93). They arise during the embryonic stage of female development when the uterus and the upper part of the vagina are formed by the coming together of two tubes, called the 'mullerian ducts'. Where this process is incomplete an abnormally shaped uterus (and sometimes also an anatomically abnormal vagina) can occur. Why this process does not always complete is usually unknown and, indeed, few women may be aware of a defect as it seldom gives trouble. As the ovaries develop independently of the uterus and vagina in the embryo there is no reason they should be affected.

More abnormalities than would be expected of the cervix, uterus and vagina have, however, been found in the daughters of women who were given high doses of oestrogens in early pregnancy to try to treat threatened miscarriage. This is the notorious DES or diethylstilboestrol syndrome, which in addition to having an association with different anatomical abnormalities of the genital tract has in some cases been found to have led to the rare 'clear cell' cancer of the vagina. As a consequence, high-dose synthetic oestrogens are no longer used in the treatment of threatened miscarriage.

Malformations are on a spectrum of mild and inconsequential to severe, needing surgery, especially when the anatomical shape of the vagina is also affected. Generally, where the vagina is blocked by malformation (see chapter 10, pages 139, 160), or where the uterus is significantly distorted from the norm, correction is possible and thought necessary as there is a clear link with infertility, recurrent miscarriage and premature labour.

The commonest abnormal uterine shape for which corrective surgery is attempted is where the joining of the mullerian ducts is not exact, producing a septate or a bicornuate uterus (see Figure 6 overleaf). In this situation it is easy to imagine that implantation of the embryo may be affected. Where only one side develops (unicornuate), or on the other extreme, where there are two of everything (didelphys), no operation is usually needed at all unless the presence of two vaginas causes coital problems and requires correction (AFS Classification, 1988).

Fibroids

Fibroids originate as benign tumours of the uterine smooth muscle wall (myometrium). They are common and are discussed separately later on in this chapter (see pages 89-96).

Figure 6 Diagrams of some uterine abnormalities

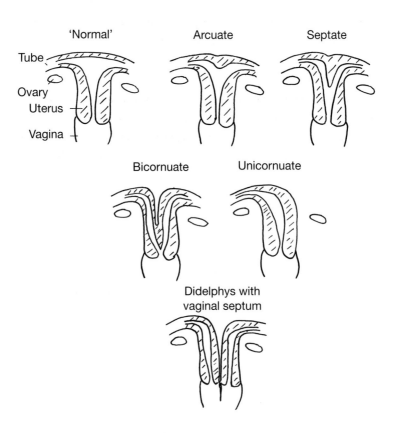

Adenomyosis

Adenomyosis is an invasion by the endometrium (uterine lining) into the myometrium and, again, is discussed later on in this chapter (section V).

Problems associated with the endometrium

Implantation

The normal uterine lining, the endometrium, changes during the menstrual cycle in response to hormonal stimulation. This stimulation is provided by the 'pituitary-ovarian hormonal axis', which is described in chapter 9.

There are three phases of the menstrual cycle, designed to prepare the uterus for the reception and nurture of a fertilised egg ('ovum'). These are the menstrual phase; the proliferative phase (also known as the follicular phase), which occurs before ovulation; and the secretory (or 'luteal') phase, which occurs after ovulation and is the phase during which implantation takes place (see chapter 9, pages 108-10).

Given the complex underlying mechanisms, it is logical to consider attributing some reproductive failures to failure of implantation, and this possibility has been much researched. However, few definitive answers have been found and no routine tests are available at present to look at implantation and its normality, or abnormality, that could be used to help the doctor make a definite clinical diagnosis of implantation failure in a patient.

Hormone imbalance

Hormone imbalance (discussed in detail in chapter 9) may lead to disruption of endometrial growth and function and to possible failure of implantation.

Auto-immune problems

'Killer T' cells in the woman's blood have been cited as a cause of implantation failure and/or very early miscarriage and I am aware that investigation and active therapy using steroids and lymphocyte transfusion is being offered in some units (chapter 10, page 185, 190; and chapter 8, page 73). However, the current scientific consensus worldwide is that further research is needed. At present, there is no scientifically valid evidence for such treatment. Patients should therefore be wary of being submitted to investigation or treatment for killer T cells unless this is as part of a valid scientific study.

Other auto-immune conditions including systemic lupus erythematosus (SLE), and the presence of high levels of anti-cardiolipid and anti-phospholipid antibodies have also been linked to early reproductive failure, possibly due to implantation having been affected (see chapter 10, page 185).

Infection

Organisms, such as the mycobacterium that causes tuberculosis (TB), can infect the endometrium. The organisms in such a case are spread internally from entry at another site in the body such as the respiratory tract. TB in the uterus causes total atrophy (wasting) and adhesions of the endometrial lining.

The other route of entry for infection to the uterus and tubes (upper genital tract) is directly upwards spread from the ever-open passage (lower genital tract) of vulva to vagina and then cervix. However, during the reproductive phase of life in particular, these organs have some protective mechanisms. These include the lips (labia) of the vulva and cervical mucus, which act as mechanical barriers, and the acidity of the vagina, which provides a very hostile environment. This ensures that the uterine cavity is normally sterile. However, infection may ascend the lower genital tract directly, entering the uterus following childbirth or iatrogenically during investigations in the area, at operation or when an IUCD (intrauterine contraceptive device) is inserted, for example.

Sexually transmitted infections such as chlamydia and gonorrhoea can ascend into the uterus via the vagina and cervix after coitus but usually pass on from it to affect the fallopian tubes rather than the uterus itself. Pyometra (infection of the endometrium) can, however, also occur, with the body's inflammatory reaction to the presence of infection possibly leading to adhesion formation and atrophy of the endometrial lining and consequent amenorrhoea (no periods). In this case, the damage can be such that, although hormone control is normal, the endometrial lining of the uterus is unable to form. There is therefore nothing to slough off at menstruation (see chapter 9, pages 108-10) and produce a period.

Asherman's syndrome

Asherman's syndrome can occur after excessive curettage (an operation to scrape out the endometrium), leading to adhesions inside the uterus and wasting of its lining. Again, damage is such that the endometrial lining does not reform and periods do not come, although some women may still experience cyclic abdominal pains.

Polyps

Polyps are small, tongue-like gatherings of endometrium. They are sometimes observed during uterine investigations. Unless large in size (10 mm+) and therefore capable of impairing implantation, they are considered of little significance in causing infertility.

Uterine factor diagnosis

History

A history of recurrent miscarriage, and/or severe dysmenorrhoea (excessive pain with periods) and/or very heavy periods (menorrhagia), may suggest your uterine muscles (myometrium) are abnormal in shape. On the other hand, if you have a history of infections, past curetting operations with abnormalities in your menstrual cycle (amenorrhoea especially), and/or recurrent failure of implantation at IVF, an abnormality in the lining of your uterus (endometrium) may be implicated.

Physical examination

'Bimanual pelvic examination' (see chapter 6) may reveal hitherto undetected anatomical abnormalities in the vagina and also in the shape of the uterus. The presence of hard pelvic masses together with an irregular-shaped uterus suggests fibroids.

Commonly used specific investigations

Abdominal and pelvic ultrasound

Abdominal ultrasound can be useful for examining the pelvic contents including the uterine wall shape and for masses such as fibroids. It is also possible, especially using vaginal ultrasound, to study the endometrial lining, its dimensions and growth (changes in thickness) accurately at different times of the cycle and also to see whether any polyps are present and to measure their size.

Pelvic ultrasound can also be used to test 'tubal patency' (whether the fallopian tubes are passable by egg and sperm) after the injection of fluid into the uterine cavity. This is known as 'hystero-contrast sonography' (HyCoSy, see page 84).

X-rays

A hysterosalpingogram (HSG) is arguably the commonest initial test used in the pelvic region in infertility. It is usually used to investigate the fallopian tubes at the same time as the uterus. An iodine-based dye is injected via the cervix. This outlines the uterine cavity shape on the X-ray monitor (hysterogram). It can be a bit uncomfortable (like bad period pains). Despite this, it is not usual practice to give more than at the most a mild analgesic, such as you might use for dysmenorrhoea. Anaesthesia is not needed. Antibiotic cover is given sometimes prophylactically or where past pelvic infection is thought to have occurred pre-procedure and for some three days afterwards. The procedure should not be performed if active pelvic infection is suspected.

Laparoscopy

Laparoscopy is described fully in the tubal section of this chapter (see page 82) as it is not generally used as a specific test of uterine function alone but as the final part of the overall utero-tubo-peritoneal investigation process that contributes to the fertility profile. Suffice to say here, it requires general anaesthesia and that a fine telescope is introduced into the abdomen via a cut usually made in the upper margin of your umbilicus (belly button). This can be up to 1 cm in length depending on the diameter of the scope. The outside of the uterus and any related masses can be evaluated as part of an overall check of the organs in the pelvis and very minor problems may be treated there and then.

Endometrial biopsy

Very small pieces of the endometrial lining can be sampled via the cervix, in outpatients or in the operating theatre, using a spoon-shaped instrument called a curette that can scrape or suck out parts of the endometrial lining. This procedure is what is known as a D&C (dilatation and curettage). Endometrial washing can also achieve the same effect. Samples obtained are then sent for laboratory examination.

Depending on the time in the menstrual cycle, the appearance of the endometrial lining alters. By timing this procedure to the second half of your cycle it is thereby possible to see whether ovulation has happened and that the secretory (or luteal) phase has commenced. This means the normality of the luteal phase can then also be investigated, although in this case serial sampling may be needed. This latter is clearly impractical for most women and there is always the chance of disturbing a very early implanting embryo.

Endometrial biopsy was at one stage the most frequently used test in infertility. It is now seldom used; hormone 'assays' and 'ultrasound follicle tracking' have replaced it for ovulation problems (see chapter 9). Curettage may, however, still be a useful method of removing polyps.

If the underlying endometrial inflammatory process (called endometritis) is thought to be caused by infection such as TB, samples can be taken similarly from the endometrium and sent for 'culture and sensitivity' (C&S – that is, infecting organisms such as bacteria, are encouraged to grow in laboratory conditions and can then be identified and destruction-tested first against antibiotics in vitro).

Hysteroscopy

In this procedure, often combined with laparoscopy for diagnostic purposes, a fine telescope is passed via the cervix, usually again under general anaesthesia. The uterine cavity is distended by a gas or a liquid so that its internal lining shape, including the openings of the fallopian tubes, can be inspected and endometrial samples taken.

Certain treatments, including polypectomy (removal of polyps), submucus myomectomy (removal of fibroids when they have grown into the uterine cavity – see page 93), and rectifying congenital uterine cavity shape defects can be carried out using the larger 'resecting operating hysteroscope'.

Pelvic MRI

Pelvic MRI (an expensive procedure) may be used in rare cases where there is doubt about the diagnosis. It has been found definitive for fibroids, adenomyosis (see pages 104-6), and uterine congenital abnormalities.

Uterine factor treatment

Problems associated with the myometrium

Congenital abnormalities

Some congenital abnormalities can be treated with a 'utriculoplasty' (plastic-surgery type) operation. Its use will depend on the type of abnormality and the realistic chances and practical value of making the uterus more anatomically normal. As it is a major procedure associated with potential problems, it is vital that the decision to use it is based on a sound knowledge of past reproductive history and on properly conducted and appropriate diagnostic investigations.

Except where the genital tract is blocked or the woman has a history of recurrent reproductive failures (see chapter 10, page 190), it is often hard to envisage how such major treatment may enhance the chances of conception other than through a placebo effect. The potential side effects may well outweigh possible benefits. Indeed, in some cases, such as congenital absence of the uterus, a surgical solution may be impossible and the only hope for a couple in having their totally own genetic child would be with the help of IVF and a surrogate mother's uterus.

Utriculoplasty operations are performed either by opening the abdomen or from below via the cervix, using a 'resecting hysteroscope'. If the latter approach is used, a camera is usually attached to the scope eyepiece and the operative looks at a TV screen, performing the operation remotely from the images provided on it. Whichever method is used, the aim is to remove any obstructions and normalise the shape, preserving uterine volume as much as is possible. After such operations it is advisable to refrain from trying to conceive for three months or so to allow the uterus and endometrial lining to heal.

Fibroids
Fibroids are discussed later in this chapter (see pages 89-96).

Adenomyosis
There is no validated treatment for adenomyosis that preserves fertility (see pages 104-6).

Problems associated with the endometrium

Implantation
Just as there is no definitive test for implantation problems as the clear cause of infertility, there is no proven treatment. Implantation problems may, however, be suspected with recurrent early miscarriage (chapter 10, page 185). Low dose aspirin can then be used under the rationale that it may improve uterine blood flow. The jury is still out as to its efficacy.

Hormone imbalance
If hormone imbalance is suspected (although absolute proof is invariably absent), the treatment of choice is 'ovarian stimulation' (see chapter 9).

Auto-immune problems
Auto-immune problems can reasonably be considered where recurrent miscarriage is the presenting symptom, or where very early miscarriages are suspected (see chapter 10, page 185). These include women known to suffer from systemic lupus erythematosus (SLE), or where routine tests show highly positive levels of anti-cardiolipin and antiphospholipid antibody levels. Low dose aspirin and heparin (which both thin the blood) can be used with good effect (see chapter 10, page 189).

As part of the 'killer T' cell story, steroids and lymphocyte transfusions are being prescribed by some specialists. These are costly, potentially problematic treatments with no proven scientific basis. At present, as I have said earlier, the consensus overall is that they should not be used except as part of an ethically approved placebo-controlled scientific trial, under regulatory authority approval, so be sure this is the case if you are offered these treatments and remember you can refuse to be part of such a trial.

Infection

It is most important to prevent infective organisms invading the reproductive system in at-risk situations for sexually transmitted disease. In such times, avoid coitus or always use a condom. However, if infection does occur, early diagnosis and antibiotic treatment are essential to try to prevent, or at the very least minimise, inflammatory pelvic damage. If worried, and do not forget that women may be symptom-free, this can best be effected by early emergency attendance for advice at your GP or STD clinic. Partner tracing is an important part of such a process.

Where the cause of the infection is systemic (a generalised infection spread via the body systems, such as TB), the treatment appropriate to the disease may occasionally help the endometrium start to function again. But, if periods have stopped ('amenorrhoea') as a result of the infection and the amenorrhoea persists after treatment, it may be necessary to prime the endometrial lining by taking oestrogens followed by progesterone tablets. This mimics the menstrual cycle hormones artificially and can get the endometrium growing again.

Asherman's syndrome

Treatment for Asherman's syndrome involves breaking down the internal uterine adhesions using a resecting hysteroscope. Following this procedure an inert intra-uterine contraceptive device (IUCD) is temporarily inserted to keep the uterine cavity open and prevent the adhesions reforming. This is usually kept in situ for up to three months, during which time oestrogens and progesterone are prescribed to promote endometrial growth.

Polyps

Polyps can be removed by curettage with or without hysteroscopic direct vision, but this needs to be done only if they are over 10 mm or causing symptoms such as heavy painful periods.

Prognosis

Uterine congenital abnormalities

In general, if you have a significant congenital uterine abnormality such as a septate or bicornuate uterus you are at higher risk of having miscarriages, premature labour and lower pregnancy rates. But, where the abnormality in shape is trivial, fecundity (the ability to achieve a live birth within one menstrual cycle) should not be affected at all and be equivalent to any fertile couple.

A septate uterus is the commonest reason for surgery. As stated at the start of this chapter, uterine malformations such as a septate uterus may develop at the time the organ is formed in the embryo if the two tubes (mullerian ducts) come together inexactly and the opposing walls do not break down properly when the uterine cavity is formed.

The septum is made up principally of fibrous tissue, with little or no uterine muscle (myometrium). Its blood supply is very poor and therefore normal endometrium uterine lining is unlikely to be formed on it. Implantation attempts at this site are therefore likely to fail.

Removal of the 'septum' by 'wedge resection utriculoplasty' is often very successful, decreasing miscarriage rates from some 80% to only 17% and increasing live births from only 18% to 91%.

Fibroids

See later on in this chapter (pages 89-96).

Adenomyosis

See later on in this chapter (pages 104-106).

Implantation failure/hormone imbalance

There is no test to confirm that infertility is caused by either implantation failure or hormone imbalance so treating these theoretical problems is hard to justify. No therapy to date has been shown to be better than doing nothing or giving a placebo.

Infection

Although the inflammatory process caused by an invading organism is usually halted by appropriate medication, the prognosis for fertility may still be poor. This is particularly true in TB where it may have been in the body for some time (chronic). In this situation, and especially with ascending STD infections such as chlamydia and gonorrhoea, tubal function will often also have been damaged. Additionally, the body's attempts at self-repair can result in adhesions forming in the uterus, similar to those in Asherman's syndrome, which compounds the problem.

Asherman's syndrome

Amenorrhoea may continue to persist after hormone treatment, even if uterine cavity adhesions are dealt with adequately and the tubes not affected. Re-establishing proper menstruation and an endometrium that is receptive to fertilised egg implantation can be achieved only in some 10% of women.

Polyps

Whether to treat or not, is the question, especially for an asymptomatic woman embarking on IVF. The present feeling is that polyps are unlikely in themselves to affect prognosis, but if they are large, it is better to remove them.

* * *

Personal Comment

> *It is difficult to use specific therapies if there are no tests to prove what the problem is in the first place. Implantation failure is one example of this. It is cited as a major excuse for lack of success, particularly following ovulation induction*

and IVF, despite little evidence at present to back up such claims. Many infertile couples are desperate and exploitable and will grasp at any straw, so please keep in mind that the risks of many treatments may outweigh the benefits and only those that have been scientifically validated for your problem are right for you. Just as operating on trivial uterine congenital abnormalities is questionable, the 'killer T' cell story is one of many that illustrates clearly the need for scientific proof before you embark on unproven and expensive diagnostic tests and potentially dangerous therapy.

SECTION II: PROBLEMS WITH THE FALLOPIAN TUBES

Anatomy and function

There is normally a pair of fallopian tubes. They extend outwards from their respective sides, left and right, of the uterus ('cornual areas', see Figure 5, page 63), sideways for some 7-8 cm towards the ovaries, starting intra-murally (within the uterine wall) and ending in a number of delicate finger like projections, the 'fimbriae'. They are not simple tubes but have secretory functions and are muscular structures lined with delicate cells with projecting hairs, or 'cilia', which by beating in one direction or another can help to transport sperm and egg.

The main functions of the fallopian tubes are to help the sperm reach the newly released egg which they do in a number of ways, including muscle contractions, beating the cilia and producing fluid to swim in. The fallopian tubes then transport the newly fertilised ovum slowly towards the uterus, retaining it until it has reached a stage in development (blastocyst) where it can be released into the uterus for implantation (5–6 days) (see chapter 2, page 6).

Main reasons for reproductive difficulty associated with the fallopian tubes

General

Any circumstances in the fallopian tubes that could interfere with transport of the sperm, gametes or newly fertilised egg, or with the mechanism by which the egg is picked up by the fimbriae (the 'ovum pick-up mechanism'), is likely to have a major effect on the chances of achieving a successful pregnancy. However, as long as one tube is intact and able to function properly, conception is still possible, although the likelihood may be reduced.

Absence of fallopian tube(s)

The fallopian tubes, like the uterus, are formed from the mullerian ducts during early embryo stage (completed after seven weeks as before then there is no differentiation between male and female). Any disruption in this process in the embryo can cause tubal malformations.

Total absence of both tubes is rare; less rare is when just one tube develops. This often occurs when only one side of the uterus develops ('unicornuate uterus'). A variation of this is when a tube may also only partially develop on the same or opposite side leaving a stump or a portion with no communication to the uterus. More commonly, the cause of an absent tube or tubes is 'iatrogenic'(the term used when the doctor has caused it directly or indirectly) because of surgical intervention, perhaps a sterilisation operation or surgery to deal with a badly infected or a ruptured tube as may follow ectopic pregnancy (pregnancy in the tube).

Direct or indirect damage

Ascending infection

Eighty-five per cent of cases of damage to the fallopian tubes are the result of infection. The incidence of tubal damage found in women with infertility is on the increase. It varies from around 20% in parts of Europe to over 50% in sub-Saharan Africa.

Ascending infection – that is, infection introduced via the cervix – is the main direct cause. The principal organisms are chlamydia and gonorrhoea, both of which are sexually transmitted. Other organisms can enter the uterus/tubes directly, for example during a complicated delivery or because of unhygienic practices at or after birth.

The damage may be direct or indirect. The presence of infective organisms will initiate the body's natural defence mechanism – an inflammatory reaction. The body's repair efforts may in turn lead to blockage of the tubes. Even if the blockage is not complete, the cilia may be damaged and cease to function.

Often both tubes are affected. The infective process can extend from the tube into the whole of the pelvis, involving all the organs of reproduction (peri-tubal-ovarian region). This is called pelvic-inflammatory disease (PID). The body's response to such infection is to form adhesions to confine it inside a wall of tissue. The result can be that even if the tubes are not blocked, the ovum pick-up mechanism (see Figure 7 overleaf) may be prevented from functioning properly, stopping for instance the sperm meeting the egg or the egg from being picked up by the tube. These adhesions can remain and may cause problems long after the infection has disappeared or become dormant.

It bears repeating that if there appears to be such an acute attack, you may feel very sick and have symptoms of pain and tenderness in the abdomen and pelvis with a smelly, possibly blood-stained vaginal discharge or, conversely you may have no symptoms at all. If you or your partner have any suspicions you should ask your doctor or an STD clinic to arrange tests for this. Diagnosis will be based on swabs taken from the genital region of both you and your partner, but the result may be negative; some infecting organisms are hard to grow.

Non-ascending infection
As with the uterus, the tubes are not immune to diseases of the whole body, such as TB, that can affect many organs. Infections can also be introduced inadvertently or already be there, stirred up from a quiescent

Figure 7 Diagrams of the tubo-ovarian pickup mechanism

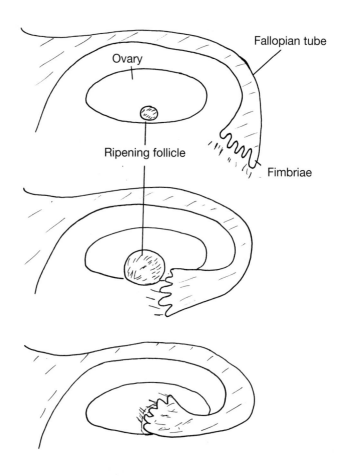

(dormant, inactive) state and propelled directly into the tubal area. This can occur during a tubal function test such as an HSG or a pelvic operation, such as surgery on the fallopian tubes, or even as a result of ovum (egg) collection at IVF. It may also happen with surgical intervention for an ectopic pregnancy or its 'sequilae' (after effects).

Infection causing PID can also spread from nearby organs such as the bowel, when bacteria present in the gut are released into the abdominal ('peritoneal') cavity. This may occur with a ruptured appendix. Ovarian cyst complications, operations on the ovaries, aspirating fluid from a cyst, especially endometriotic (see page 101) with a needle, and removal of cysts can all invoke the same potentially damaging but nevertherless life-saving (on occasion) natural body inflammatory repair mechanism.

Endometriosis

Endometriosis may also prevent pick-up of the egg by the fimbriae (the 'ovum pick-up mechanism') if it has caused adhesions (see page 97).

Mechanical problems (iatrogenic)

In addition to situations where the tubes have been removed because of infection or ectopic pregnancy, many couples now elect to have this done when they feel their family is complete. Sterilisation in the woman is a more final option than in the man, usually involving clipping or tying both tubes with or without removing a portion of each via a laparoscope. It may be acceded to even when the woman is still young (under 30). However, not infrequently nowadays, social circumstances change and a child is again desired, resulting in a request for the now regretted tubal sterilisation operation to be reversed.

Tubal factor diagnosis

General

Many of the functions of the fallopian tubes that are vital for the process of conception cannot be tested. The most important of these that can are patency (the tubes being 'open') and to some extent movement at the fimbrial end and the anatomical mechanism by which the fimbriae pick up the egg (the 'ovum pick-up mechanism').

History

The infertile couple's history is often unhelpful. If, however, you are aware that you or your partner has had pelvic infection in the past, the ravages caused to pelvic organs by ascending STD infection may be hidden. Pain on intercourse ('deep dyspareunia') and more non-specific symptoms, such as worse than usual dysmenorrhoea (pain at period time), menorrhagia or the opposite amenorrhoea, may, however, indicate present, or past, pelvic infection or utero-tubal adhesions. A history of the last conception resulting in an ectopic pregnancy or an infected miscarriage requiring evacuation under antibiotic cover, a difficult vaginal birth, a vaginal operative delivery, puerperal infection with infected smelly lochia (the blood-stained discharge after birth) may all be clues to raise the possibility of a tubal factor in women with secondary infertility.

Physical examination

There may be very few, or no, physical signs. With an acute infection, body temperature is generally raised. The woman's abdomen may be tender and 'bimanual vaginal examination' be painful. The doctor may be able to feel enlarged fallopian tubes and/or tender masses at the side of the uterus that indicate infection or adhesions.

Tubal patency tests

Some fertility centres insist on serologically screening all patients for chlamydia as part of routine management for all tests of tubal patency as this is the most common cause of STD tubal infections and often hidden. Routine antibiotic cover is frequently given while invasive tubal function tests are carried out.

Laparoscopy

Pelvic disease involving the tubes and the ovum pick-up mechanism is diagnosed best by laparoscopy plus dye injection. Under anaesthetic, following the insertion of CO_2 (carbon dioxide) gas through a needle (verres) to create a pneumoperitoneum (blow up the abdomen with gas) so that the organs can be seen properly and inspected, a viewing telescope (laparoscope) is inserted. This is passed through a small cut, usually sited in the top margin of the navel with the entrance to the abdomen made with the help of a trochar and cannula (spike and tube). This allows the gynaecologist to inspect the pelvic contents and to move the tubes and ovaries around. Dye can be injected via the cervix to test patency (that the tubes are 'open'). The spill of the dye is then seen directly at the ends of the tubes if the tubes are open. Other potential 'pathology' in the uterus, ovaries and rest of the pelvis, such as adhesions, cysts, fibroids and endometriosis can be seen and evaluated.

Although at this stage such a procedure is primarily diagnostic, in some instances mild adhesions and endometriosis, small ovarian cysts and fibroids can be dealt with at the same time if you have given provisional consent in advance. It is advisable, when you are asked for consent, to enquire who will be carrying out the procedure and what their level of training/expertise is.

The procedure is not without hazard. In addition to anaesthetic problems, rare complications can occur during the procedure, even if it is done for purely diagnostic purposes. A major complication is perforation of the bowel or damage to other adjacent organs by instruments. It can also be expensive, which is important to bear in mind as there is little correlation between the procedure and the incidence of pregnancy. For this reason, while the vast majority of specialists agree that laparoscopy is the reference test (diagnostic procedure of choice) for utero-tubal-peritoneal function, some authorities recommend laparoscopy for selective infertility situations only. They suggest limiting its use to when there is a history of PID, an abnormality in other screening tests or where there is longstanding 'unexplained infertility' or suspicion of endometriosis. However, where laparoscopy is used only in this manner, much, possibly asymptomatic, that is of potential significance for fertility can be missed, especially adhesions around the tubes and endometriosis.

X-ray hysterosalpingography (HSG)

As previously mentioned (see page 70), HSG is an out-patient procedure that tests tubal patency (that the fallopian tubes are 'open'), but muscular spasm in the tubes may cause false negatives. While the site of an obstruction in a tube can be usefully pinpointed and the uterine cavity outlined, an HSG does not show the area around the outside of the tubes efficiently. Structures cannot be moved and the presence of factors like adhesions or endometriosis that are potentialy significant to normal tubal pick-up mechanism function are unlikely to be diagnosed.

HyCoSy

As I said earlier in the section about the uterus (pages 69-70) some fertility units use HyCoSy (hystero-contrast sonography) instead of HSG X-ray. Ultrasound enables the health professional carrying this procedure out to visualise the passage of fluid through the tubes. The benefits and limitations are similar as with HSG.

Falloposcopy/salpingoscopy

'Falloposcopy', or 'salpingoscopy', was introduced in an effort to visualise the inside lining of the fallopian tubes. A small telescope is introduced via the abdomen and threaded into the tube via the fimbriae at the end of the tubes, or from below via the cervix with the aid of a hysteroscope. It has not become a routine test as it is difficult to perform and most authorities, excepting a few enthusiasts, question the value of the information that the procedure provides.

Tubal insufflation tests

I am including tubal insufflation, also known as Rubin's test, solely to exclude it. The test involved carbon dioxide gas being blown through the tubes via the cervix and uterus and the sound of it 'escaping through the end of the tubes' being listened to with a stethoscope placed in the woman's groin areas. At one time it was often combined with a D&C. By now it should have been consigned to history, being inadequate and potentially dangerous. You should refuse this procedure if it is offered.

Tubal factor treatments

General

It is important to consider the function of both left and right fallopian tubes. Treatment may not be needed at all where the problem is only on one side and the other tube and its pick-up mechanisms appear normal.

Absent or incomplete tubes

There is no restorative treatment if the tubes are missing or incomplete. IVF allows the tubes to be bypassed.

Direct or indirect damage

Prevention and treatment of infection

Antibiotics are the drugs of choice in the case of 'ascending' infections (infections that have entered via the cervix) given either prophylactically or as soon after the potential infective event as can be. If possible, they should be selected specifically for the most likely infecting organism until culture results of swabs are returned from the lab, when treatment may need to be changed. However, antibiotics cannot be guaranteed to be effective in getting rid of the infection entirely. It may become chronic or almost dormant, only to flare up again on another occasion. In addition, adhesions may still form, especially if there is a delay in getting the right drug, and cause more problems than the infection itself.

Prophylactic antibiotics can be used preventatively if there is a risk of infection spreading from other organs, for example with peritonitis following appendicitis and bowel rupture.

Surgery during diagnosis

During diagnostic laparoscopy, if minor adhesions are found to be binding down patent (open) tubes, these adhesions can usually be easily and beneficially divided ('adhesiolysis') at the same time.

Formal tubal surgery

Tubal surgery, where the fallopian tubes are distorted, blocked or densely stuck down, can in many cases offer chances of pregnancy on a par with those offered by IVF. In addition, unlike IVF, if surgery cures the problem, with this comes the chance of more babies naturally without any further treatment.

Macro- and microsurgical (using magnification to see better) operations via the abdomen or through a laparoscope can both be successful given the right experience, training and facilities. Sadly, tubal surgery is a dying art in many units, but it should be available as an option in any tertiary fertility centre.

Three types of operation can be performed depending on the problem. These are: division of adhesions (salpingolysis); the re-opening of the end of tube if blocked (salpingostomy); and, where the blockage is in the tube, the removal of the blocked section and the re-joining of the ends (re-anastomosis). Unfortunately, however, while re-anastomosis may be the way forward for reversing tubal sterilisation operations, this may not be achievable in all circumstances. For example, if the tubes have been removed totally or too much has been taken away or if there has been excessive adhesion formation, surgery to rejoin them will not work. Notes of previous operations in the area may help decide what is possible, together with further tests and careful evaluation, including the help of a counsellor.

IVF

IVF is the only option now offered in many centres for tubal factor infertility. This approach can be understandable if suitable facilities for alternatives are not available or assessment suggests an attempt at reconstructive surgery would be futile. Indeed, in such circumstances, it may also be more appropriate to remove a diseased tube, especially if swollen and dilated by fluid (hydrosalpinx) or infection (pyosalpinx) first before IVF is carried out as this may improve the prognosis (chances of success).

Prognosis

General

Pregnancies have been recorded after both HSG and diagnostic laparoscopy utero-tubal investigations in up to 10% of cases. Cleaning out, or flushing through, the tubes is cited as the reason but it is hard to envisage this is correct scientifically. A placebo effect (see chapter 5, page 26) is the likely cause.

Absence of tubes

If one tube is normal, operation on the other is not warranted and may lead to problems on the normal side. If the fallopian tubes are missing on both sides, no corrective treatment is possible. Prognosis in terms of conception is zero without IVF.

Direct or indirect damage

Infection

Most antibiotics, if appropriately chosen and with timely adequate administration, can be expected to cure an acute infection fully or to help in prophylaxis (preventative) situations, but less when there is a chronic infection. If a hidden infection is left untreated and affects both fallopian tubes, the inflammatory response of itself may result in a woman becoming or remaining infertile unless she has surgery or IVF.

Surgery

Data relating to the success of tubal surgery are hard to pin down. Figures quoted in the scientific literature for subsequent pregnancy suffer from selectivity and lack of consistency as to whether one or both tubes was affected or treated. In prognostic terms, the results of surgery need to be compared with the incidence of pregnancy from IVF per cycle started. This averages in the latest available (2004) ESHRE European multi-national figures a success rate of approximately 31% per transfer (see chapter 11, page 242).

The efficacy of tubal surgery depends on how badly damaged the tube itself, or the peri-tubal-ovarian region, is. Where mild to moderate adhesions around the tubes are divided and there is no evidence of further tubal disease, fecundity rates (the ability to achieve a pregnancy within one month) can be normal, although, as with all tubal surgery, ectopic pregnancy rates are higher than normal. Where more major adhesions are treated (salpingolysis), reported figures indicate an overall intrauterine pregnancy rate of around 26%. For this reason, if pregnancy has not started after six months, follow-up is needed, with a second laparoscopy, and IVF may possibly be recommended.

When the tubes are blocked in the mid part, 're-anastomosis' may be particularly successful, depending on the age of the woman, both for reversing sterilisation operations (up to 60% achieve pregnancy) and for blockages from other clauses (more than 55% achieve pregnancy). However, if the tube(s) appear dilated and filled with fluid ('balloon-like hydrosalpinx') due to blockage at or near the fimbrial end, and the cilia and/or fimbriae have been destroyed, the chances of achieving a successful uterine pregnancy by unblocking the end (salpingostomy) are very poor.

Discuss the options with great care before giving your consent to surgery and be aware of the chances of success. Whatever surgical procedure is carried out, it is important to realise that the risk of a subsequent ectopic (tubal) pregnancy is considerably increased (relative risk 20%). This compares with a much lower relative risk of 2% with IVF.

Surgery where endometriosis is present

See page 101 in this chapter.

Surgery for iatrogenic-induced blockage

Reversal of sterilisation should always be explored before embarking on IVF. If the conditions are right, it can increase the chance of pregnancy to a level equal to a fertile couple's each month.

* * *

Personal Comment

For most couples, finding a cause for ongoing infertility transcends all other considerations. Without laparoscopy the incidence of 'unexplained infertility' doubles. This must not be forgotten when you are discussing with your doctor which tests of tubal function to undergo. Remember too that much damage is still caused by operations and ascending infection despite antibiotics being readily available. The incidence of this as a cause of tubal-factor infertility is increasing. If this trend is to be reversed worldwide, better awareness is needed of the damage infection can cause, together with avoidance of risky intercourse and the consistent use of optimal birthing practices. IVF has undoubtedly transformed the prognosis for women with tubal-factor infertility, but there is still a place to try surgery first in selected situations.

* * *

SECTION III: FIBROIDS

What are fibroids?

Fibroids are tumours containing a mixture of smooth muscle and fibrous tissue. They arise initially from the muscle wall of the uterus and are the most common benign tumour found in women. Their incidence varies with age. For years, the figure of some 25% has been quoted in menopausal women. Some 1-2% are found in pregnant women; during the pregnancy they may grow, shrink or degenerate due to interference with the blood supply.

Fibroids may be single or multiple. They may be very small but can grow extremely large (in excess of a term pregnancy). They can become detached from the uterus. These are known as 'parasitic' as they get their subsequent blood supply from a non-uterine source. They have arterial and venous blood supply from the vessels supplying the uterus. Malignant cancerous change is extremely rare. It occurs, if ever, in predominately older women in fewer than one in a hundred of cases. They are called 'sarcomas' rather than the more familiar carcinoma as they come from connective tissue (muscle and blood vessels) rather than epithelial tissues.

Why may fibroids be important in infertility?

It is not always easy to justify the finding of fibroids as a sole cause for a woman's infertility problem. Only 2–3% are thought significant. However, they can possibly affect fertility mechanically by growing in the uterine wall (see Figure 8 opposite) from where they invariably start (intramural fibroids) and then distort it. This may in turn affect implantation or block the cervix and fallopian tubes.

Fibroids can grow inwards into the uterine cavity ('submucus' development) and obstruct it, or outwards into the abdomen ('serous' development) and obstruct tubal movement and/or the ovum pick-up mechanism. They are often found in combination with endometriosis, which is not a good sign for fertility.

Causes

What causes fibroids to develop is unknown. They can run in families, and are found more frequently in black women than caucasians, often in conjunction with endometriosis. High oestrogen levels are linked to their presence. They are more common in diabetics and in women who have never been pregnant; the risk of fibroids developing later on is halved after just two pregnancies.

Diagnosis

History

In younger woman fibroids may cause no symptoms. They most commonly come to light by chance during investigations for utero-tubal factors or during a pregnancy. The commonest associated symptom is menorrhagia (heavy periods), which may give rise to anaemia. Sometimes there will be a feeling of fullness and pressure. Complications such as torsion (twisting) or degeneration may cause acute abdominal pain.

Physical examination

Nothing may be felt on examination but, depending on size site and number, a typical hard, round mass may be felt distorting the uterus

Figure 8 Commonest sites of fibroids

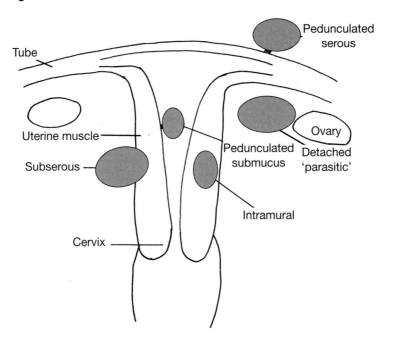

or may be found to arise separately out of the pelvis on bimanual or abdominal examination by the doctor.

Tests

Pelvic ultrasound is the best and most cost-effective method for formal evaluation of suspected fibroids. It can help differentiate a fibroid from other common masses that may be found in the same area. These are, most commonly, trapped wind (flatus), a fetus, fat and ovarian cysts.

Ultrasound is also useful for estimating the size and number, and their impact on the uterus. It allows health professionals to review the situation non-invasively from time to time.

Plain abdominal X-ray

Plain abdominal X-ray will show fibroids only if there is calcification (the so-called 'womb stone'), but distortion of the uterus noted at HSG may suggest they are present.

Hysteroscopy

Hysteroscopy can detect the submucus type of fibroid and those in the uterine wall that are impinging and distorting the uterine cavity. It can help to differentiate them from a large intrauterine polyp (a nodule of the endometrial lining).

MRI (magnetic resonance imaging)

If fibroids are located 'intra-murally', they can be confused with 'focal adenomyosis' (see page 106). MRI will help differentiate one from the other. This is important as fibroids can be removed at operation. Adeno-myosis cannot unless hysterectomy is performed, which in an infertile woman trying to conceive would be a disaster.

Treatments

Myomectomy

Myomectomy via an abdominal incision is the commonest approach in infertile women if an intramural or serous-sited fibroid(s) is reckoned to be over 5 cm in diameter or multiple, but this is not without hazard. It is major surgery requiring skilled technique and experience. The operation can be difficult, complications may arise, including haemorrhage necessitating hysterectomy, and pelvic adhesion formation may follow. Fibroids will recur in up to 15%. Women in an infertile relationship should therefore not agree to myomectomy unless it appears that fibroids really are contributing to childlessness.

Uncomplicated serous-sited fibroids can also be removed sometimes laparoscopically via a small abdominal incision; for submucus fibroids, operative hysteroscopy will allow resection and removal via the cervix as this avoids opening the uterine cavity to gain access.

Hysterectomy

Hysterectomy is not usually relevant to an infertile woman but, where no further pregnancies are desired and periods are very heavy and painful (menorrhagic), it may be worth considering removal of the uterus. This is technically easier than a myomectomy – it is easier to remove the uterus than to try to restore it. A progesterone loaded intrauterine coil (IUCD) may be an alternative to buy time instead of a hysterectomy in this situation.

X-ray embolisation

X-ray embolisation is a new approach that can be useful for single large fibroids. The size of the fibroid is shrunk (degeneration) by interfering with the arterial blood supply feeding it. The radiologist passes a tube through the woman's arteries to the fibroid from an appropriately placed vessel on the woman's skin and injects a substance (sclerosant) to block the feeding artery at the entrance (pedicle) to the fibroid.

Medical/hormonal

Medical and hormonal methods of attempting to shrink fibroids usually use GnRH (gonadotrophin releasing hormone) agonists. The idea is to cut down oestrogen levels (E2) that promote and sustain the fibroids' growth. These drugs interfere with FSH production in the pituitary gland that stimulates E2 production (see chapter 9, pages 108-10). Ovulation and periods stop and the fibroids shrink. The GnRH agonist is usually given over a 3-6 month period, depending on response.

Other drugs called GnRH antagonists have also been used by some doctors before myomectomy to try to make the surgery easier. The maximum effect is seen by 14 days. The antagonist is therefore quicker to use than the agonist, but both are impractical as the sole treatment in infertility where time is usually of the essence.

Prognosis

When reviewing claims of success for all these treatments, it is important to remember that the relationship between fibroid presence and infertility is doubtful in many cases. Any claimed success could quite possibly therefore be as the result of a strong placebo effect.

Myomectomy

Myomectomy, either abdominally or laparoscopically, in the short term (up to six months) seems to give excellent pregnancy rates (50%+). This seems to be particularly true where the operation is relatively 'avascular' (little blood loss has occurred), a single fibroid has been easily removed and there was no necessity to go into the uterine cavity to aid its removal.

If pregnancy has not started within six months, further consideration is, however, needed. This is because there is the possibility of recurrence (15%) or of further growth if inaccessibility has precluded removing all fibroids present. Additionally, the situation may have been made worse by operative adhesion formation after the original myomectomy. Laparoscopy, with tubal surgery to follow if necessary, may then be needed.

Embolisation

Embolisation to date has not been performed in sufficient comparative trials to judge its prognosis compared with other treatments. It can cause fibroids to shrink but not to disappear totally with any speed. The distorting effect the fibroid was producing may continue as its outer capsule may remain. Surgery may be needed later to remove this. A year interval is recommended after embolisation before attempting to conceive.

Medical/hormonal treatment

GnRH agonists may eventually 'shrink' some fibroids (30-60%). Hot flushes and amenorrhoea occur during such lengthy therapy and reversible bone loss (osteoporosis) can develop. There is no chance of pregnancy during the time on treatment and usually for some two to three months afterwards. Following the end of therapy, fibroid growth can increase rapidly if they are not removed.

Personal Comment

Many women have fibroids and they may often be treated unnecessarily. However, when their position or sheer size appears to be a factor preventing successful conception, removal is best. Depending on size, number and site, often an open operation with abdominal incision is less technically challenging than struggling with the increasingly common 'keyhole' laparoscopic approach. Both require special training and instruments. Whatever approach is used, it is important that your surgeon understands that body structures close to the fibroid(s) must be preserved as much as pos-

sible and that any possible adhesion formation must be minimised. It may be better to leave some small or inaccessible fibroids in situ than to jeopardise reproductive chances further.

SECTION IV: ENDOMETRIOSIS

What is endometriosis?

Endometriosis is defined as the presence of tissue in sites in the body outside the uterus ('ectopic') with a microscopic appearance similar to the uterine lining (endometrium). Like the endometrium, it is dependent on the function of ovarian hormones, especially oestrogens (see chapter 9).

It is commonly found in fertile women of reproductive age (that is, in up to one in ten), particularly in the pelvic area, but is particularly prevalent in women with infertility.

This prevalence in infertile women seems to vary between different parts of the world. It has been reported in the past (WHO, 1988) as uncommon in infertile women in Africa (affecting only 1%), in 10% of infertile women in Asia, and 6% in Europe. This obviously under-reported variation may, however, have had much to do with the availability of laparoscopy, which is needed to make a definitive diagnosis and is unlikely to reflect the present position.

The amounts of endometriosis (ectopic endometrium) vary from a few spots, which may even go unnoticed, to a large ovarian cyst filled with old blood ('endometrioma' or 'chocolate cyst'). There can be multiple large lesions which lead to the formation of extensive adhesions and thus to what is called 'frozen pelvis'.

Why may endometriosis be important in infertility?

Although commonly found in infertile women, in many cases it is hard to see a mechanical cause and effect link between the endometriosis that is seen and infertility. Indeed, some authorities feel the presence of minimal amounts alone is simply a variant of pelvic normality. It has been suggested that in minimal grade endometriosis the main problem could be that the peritoneal fluid (the fluid that naturally occurs in the abdominal cavity and bathes all the organs) may be altered by endometriosis and that this then affects fertility by altering functions such as sperm motility, fallopian tube movements, and/or sex hormone secretion in the immediate areas surrounding the reproductive organs.

It is much easier to regard endometriosis as a cause of infertility when the adhesion-forming inflammatory reaction that can occur interferes with the ovum pick-up mechanism or when an endometrioma (ovarian cyst) is found which can adversely affect ovum growth, egg quality and release.

Finally, increased miscarriage rates have also been cited by some experts but not confirmed by others.

Causes

There are a number of theories (this means we do not really know or there is no single true cause) as to why endometriosis occurs. No one alone fits the bill properly. The most popular and easiest to understand is still the suggestion, first made in 1927, that menstrual fluid passes via the tubes into the abdominal (peritoneal) cavity (retrograde menstruation) as well as out through the cervix, carrying endometrial fragments. Some of these cells implant themselves and grow in the nearby peritoneal area.

This theory fits well with the main sites in which endometriosis is found in infertility (see Figure 9, page 99). These are on the ovary, in the peri-tubular area and in the cul-de-sac area between the back of the uterus, cervix and rectum (called the 'Pouch of Douglas'). However, it is not the whole story. It is thought that all women who menstruate have retrograde menstruation, but not all have endometriosis.

Endometriosis can more rarely be found in many other parts of the body, including the eye, chest and tonsils. Other theories as to cause include: spread by blood and the lymphatic system; genetic/inheritance; the presence of developmental embryonic rests (during embryonic development some cells that are eventually to form and function as endometrium in the reproductive years fail to migrate to the right place); metaplasia (one tissue changing into another); and immunological factors.

Diagnosis

History

Many infertile women with endometriosis are asymptomatic. Infertility may be the only presenting complaint and when endometriosis is found it comes as a surprise. Abdomino-pelvic pain, especially associated with periods (dysmenorrhoea), can be passed off as no different from usual. In some women, however, periods become more painful than before.

Painful intercourse on deep penetration (dyspareunia) can also be a characteristic complaint (see chapter 10, page 160).

The extent of the symptoms is often inversely related to the extent of the disease – that is, the more endometriotic tissue is present, the less the symptoms. Small amounts of deep-seated endometriosis seem to be more painful. If not properly investigated, some women can be labelled in error as having irritable bowel syndrome (IBS) as the symptoms can be similar.

Physical examination

Physical examination may be negative, even with extensive lesions, or falsely positive with none. Suspicious signs on pelvic examination include tender nodules (small lumps) to the side of the vagina, a fixed retroverted (tilted backwards) uterus and a tender ovarian cyst.

Tests

Ovarian ultrasound may by chance reveal a cyst that is more opaque than usual in the ovary. Endometrial fluid, which is old blood, is thick, appearing just like 'chocolate sauce'.

Figure 9 Diagram of commonest sites of endometriosis

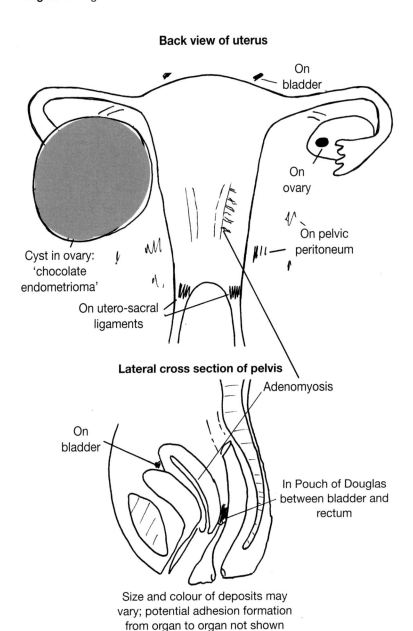

Back view of uterus

On bladder

On ovary

On pelvic peritoneum

Cyst in ovary: 'chocolate endometrioma'

On utero-sacral ligaments

Lateral cross section of pelvis

Adenomyosis

On bladder

In Pouch of Douglas between bladder and rectum

Size and colour of deposits may vary; potential adhesion formation from organ to organ not shown

Blood Ca125

Levels of a test called Ca125 can be raised but this is not specific to endometriosis and occurs in other situations, including some cancers (ovarian especially) and any other condition causing peritoneal (abdominal internal lining) irritation.

Laparoscopy

Direct visualisation by pelvic laparoscopy is the only true way of making a diagnosis. It is the gold standard but is unfortunately an operation that is not without potential complications (see opposite). This is acceptable to most when it is used in making an initial diagnosis or after long-term failure of specific therapy, but it is hard to justify repeating the procedure more than once just to monitor treatment. However, there is nothing else available for this task. Most authorities consider biopsy of lesions to confirm the diagnosis to be generally unnecessary, even though the appearance of deposits of endometriosis can vary across a wide spectrum of colours.

Classification

Laparoscopy also enables classification. This helps determine which treatment is going to be best and the potential prognosis. The main classification system in use was devised by the American Fertility Society (now the American Society for Reproductive Medicine – ASRM). It was revised in 1985. It does not count lesions outside the pelvis.

It includes four classification stages (numbered 1 to 4), varying from a few spots (stage 1) through to a completely frozen pelvis (stage 4). Combining the AFS stages into the terms mild (a few spots), moderate (lesions with mild adhesion formation), and severe (endometriomas and/or the presence of extensive adhesions) is often a more useful guide for health professionals and you as to when to treat and how.

Treatments

General

The three alternatives for dealing with intolerable pain caused by endometriosis – long-term suppression of the ovaries by drugs, pre-sacral
'neurectomy' or removal of the ovaries – are all totally inappropriate in
women wishing to conceive. Indeed, this symptom is quite rare in women
with infertility.

Surgery

Whether to treat at all where there is infertility is controversial. When
the endometriosis found is mild to moderate without anatomical distortion there is a case for doing nothing, but leaving it may carry the risk
of progression to more major pathology.

The conflict is whether removing the lesions has more than a placebo effect, especially if potential side effects are taken into account.
The majority of specialists in the field feel that, overall, if mild endometriosis is found during the initial diagnostic laparoscopy, and if
the operative is properly trained and has facilities for burning lesions
off (ablation by end coagulation or laser), then these lesions should be
treated there and then.

There is also little quarrel with removal of adhesions that affect and
distort the environment around the ovum pick-up mechanism as a way
of restoring anatomical normality. If adhesions are mild to moderate
these can also be divided during diagnostic laparoscopy.

If laparoscopy reveals severe endometriosis, the course of action is
clearer. With extensive moderate or severe (stage 3-4) adhesions, or in the
presence of a large (5 cm+) endometrioma, it is generally agreed that surgery at a later date is the way forward. The aim of this it to remove the
abnormal tissue either laparoscopically or via the abdomen. A tubal micro-
surgeon's training can be very beneficial in terms of improving the chances
of conception. Before starting, the benefits of surgery need to be weighed
up against doing nothing, adding in medical therapy first, or going to IVF.

With all operative treatments, adhesions can be created and endometriosis may return even if fully removed. If pregnancy has still not started after six months the situation needs to be reviewed, as in some 45%+ of cases thus treated, there may be further progression.

Medical/hormonal

Before the advent of GnRH agonists, and still sometimes now, the oral contraceptive pill, or androgens such as danazol, or progestogens such as medroxyprogesterone acetate, were given continuously, initially for three cycles at a time. All suppress ovarian function and consequently menstruation ceases; it is hoped endometriosis regresses. More recently GnRHa (gonadotrophin releasing hormone agonist therapy) has been used to create what is termed a pseudo-menopause. Treatment is for a maximum of six months.

Nowadays drug therapy is used as first choice only occasionally in endometriotic infertility if ablation is not possible, or to try to 'shrink' an endometrioma. Pregnancy is not possible while such treatment is ongoing, a major handicap if time is of the essence.

As previously mentioned, GnRH agonists are more often used before or after major endometriotic surgery for some three months, as an adjunct to healing. They have also been used before IVF to try to 'shrink' any small endometriomas (2-4 cm), but with little reported success.

IVF

IVF under antibiotic cover is always a possible alternative, especially if major surgery is needed for the endometriosis or the case is inoperable. For those who wish to continue with such an active approach, IVF will need to be discussed (see chapter 11, page 209-46).

Prognosis

General

The general prognosis is difficult to predict, particularly as the significance of endometriosis as a definite causative factor in infertility is unknown. It has been known to disappear spontaneously. Conversely, by five years after apparently successful removal, endometriosis will have recurred in up to 40% of women. In minimal/mild (stage 1-2) endometriosis, untreated pregnancy rates have been found to be some 8% compared to 20% in unexplained infertility.

Surgery

Laparoscopic surgical ablation in minimal/mild endometriosis has been found to give a pregnancy rate of some 27% compared with 18% of untreated, laparoscoped controls. In severe endometriosis, a surgical approach aimed at restoring the anatomy to normal has been known to achieve pregnancy success in up to 35% of women. In moderate disease this effect increases to approximately 60%.

Overall, the available data suggest an improvement in spontaneous pregnancy rates of some 30% can be expected with removal of endometriosis. This is similar to the expected placebo effect any investigations and treatment in infertility may have. The couples undergoing treatment for endometriosis have, however, not already benefited from that placebo effect chance.

Medical/hormonal

Drug treatment alone has not been found to improve fertility. Indeed, if all the stages in endometriosis as classified by the American Fertility Society (AFS) are included, in-depth comparative analysis of the scientific literature (meta-analysis) seems to show no difference in effect between medical treatment and no treatment.

IVF

With IVF, expected pregnancy rates do not appear to be affected by the presence of any stage of endometriosis despite egg quality often being poorer. There is, however, a greater danger of complications at egg collection, particularly of inducing infection, if disease is active or an endometrioma is present. Antibiotic cover is usually given.

Personal Comment

Endometriosis is commonly found in women of reproductive age. It is often but not always associated with infertility. It can be a chance finding. The main handicap to diagnosis and treatment is not being able to see what is going on. Until there is a solution to this problem, mis-diagnosis will occur and how therapy is progressing with be guesswork. Further major management difficulties include lack of knowledge about the likelihood of it remaining mild, or progressing quickly to the severe stage, or disappearing spontaneously. Whichever is to happen is pure guesswork. It seems wisest to treat it appropriately whenever it is found, whatever the grade, so long as the side effects of treatment do not lower the chances of a pregnancy occurring.

SECTION V: ADENOMYOSIS

What is adenomyosis?

Sometimes described as 'internal endometriosis', adenomyosis is the term used when endometrial glands are found growing up into the uterine muscle layer detached from the endometrial lining. It may occur throughout the uterus (diffuse) or at one focal point similar to a fibroid. Unlike endometriosis, the tissue does not appear to respond to menstrual cycle hormones.

Why may adenomyosis be important in infertility?

Adenomyosis may be part of normal uterine aging. It may contribute to the lowering of pregnancy chances as age increases by the distorting effect it may have on the uterus. This, in theory, may cause infertility or implantation problems. There are no tests to confirm these theoretical possibilities.

Causes

These are unknown. Possibly it is a physiologically normal occurrence.

Diagnosis

History

The woman is usually in her 40s. As many women over 40 now present with fertility problems adenomyosis should be considered as a potential cause of infertility in women of this age. It is often found in older women who are having hysterectomies because of menorrhagia (very heavy periods).

Physical examination

On pelvic examination the uterus will be soft and enlarged, often uniformly.

Tests

Laparoscopy
It may be suspected at diagnostic laparoscopy if the uterus appears enlarged.

MRI (magnetic resonance imaging)
This expensive test is best utilised if the differential diagnosis between adenomyosis and fibroid(s) is unclear and an operation to remove the latter is being contemplated.

Treatment and prognosis

Surgical

Surgery for adenomyosis is not usually of interest to the infertile woman desiring a baby as hysterectomy is the optimal therapy if menorrhagia is severe. Indeed, unless menstrual problems are affecting quality of life, active treatment is seldom recommended as adenomyosis may be part of the normal aging process.

Medical

GnRH agonists have been alleged to help fertility if the disease is focal (not diffuse). Data are very scant. Success has been claimed in two case reports only.

Personal Comment

Adenomyosis is more likely a phenomenon of age than a disease entity. It is commoner in older women. It is often linked to both endometriosis (being called by some, internal endometriosis) and sometimes mistaken as a fibroid. Differentiation from other conditions is important if surgery is contemplated. There is no treatment for it that preserves the chances of conception. If this is important, it may be best to leave well alone.

Chapter 9

Ovulation factors

MYTH

A regular 28-day menstrual cycle guarantees ovulation is taking place mid-cycle.

Some general facts about ovarian function and ovulation

The human female normally has two ovaries. These are situated in the pelvis (see Figures 1 and 5, pages 5 and 63) on either side of the uterus near the ends of the fallopian tubes (fimbriae). During the reproductive phase of female life, their function is to produce eggs and sex hormones. Production of sex hormones, although somewhat altered, still persists after the menopause; egg production does not. Follicular loss (follicles are the fluid-filled sacs in the ovaries containing the eggs that develop each cycle) speeds up as ovarian function declines with age.

While menstruation is a good sign, it does not guarantee ovulation has taken place. Although there are worldwide variations, failure to ovulate (anovulation) is the commonest single infertility factor (35%) found in most fertility clinics. Ovulation itself and the causes of failure to ovulate (anovulation) are better understood than any other factor in the infertility profile. This is due to our in-depth knowledge of how the menstrual cycle is controlled and the exact diagnostic tools available to investigate it. As a result, diagnosis of the cause is relatively easy, as is designing appropriate therapy. A greater degree of direct success can be anticipated for anovulation therapy than for any other fertility treatment.

The menstrual cycle and its control

It is helpful to know about the menstrual cycle and how it is controlled, to understand both this chapter and infertility in general.

Menstrual fluid contains blood, mucus and the sloughed-off lining of the uterus (endometrium). It is expelled from the uterus via the cervix into the vagina some 14 days after ovulation if pregnancy does not occur. Menstruation is usually cyclical, but only 15% of menstrual cycles will be exactly 28 days from the previous one. However, this is the length of time most often used for descriptive purposes (see Figure 10, page 111) so I also shall use it here. Days 1-5 are taken as the menstruation phase, day 14 as the day of ovulation and day 28 as the day when the cycle ends and the next menstruation and cycle begin.

Noticeable cyclic changes occur also in the cervical secretions and the breasts. Moods alter as can basal body temperatures (see Figure 11, page 117).

What happens?

I describe the menstrual cycle here in the most basic of terms only, beginning with the onset of menstruation and the brain's hypothalamic-pituitary-axis function (see Figure 12, page 121). The hypothalamus (a part of the brain) secretes a gonadotrophin-releasing hormone (GnRH), which passes via a blood (portal) vessel down to the adjacent pituitary gland (a part of the brain situated in the middle behind the eyes). This stimulates pituitary cells to produce a follicle-stimulating hormone (FSH) and luteinising hormone (LH).

This GnRH stimulation process is always working but is particularly active during menses (menstruation). It starts off the process of egg and endometrial development (the development of the inner lining of the uterus, which has a very rich blood supply) for each cycle. Pituitary FSH then stimulates the ovaries. Several of the inactive primordial follicles present in the ovary, each of which contains an immature egg, are recruited and start to develop under FSH influence (follicular development). The follicle is the fluid-filled sac containing an egg. The egg, or eggs, start to grow and mature. Usually only one follicle per cycle eventually becomes fully mature (the dominant follicle).

FSH also directs the ovary to start producing oestrogen (oestradiol, or 'E2'). Increasing amounts of E2 are then produced up until the periovular phase of the cycle (days 12-14). In the uterus, the E2 stimulates the growth of the lining (endometrium) in preparation for receiving a possible pregnancy. This is called the follicular or proliferative phase.

As E2 rises, it feeds back negatively to the hypothalamic-pituitary axis, diminishing the production of GnRH and FSH as further output of these hormones is not needed. Conversely, it also feeds back positively to the pituitary gland to stimulate more LH production. When the dominant follicle is ripe (days 12-13), there is a surge in LH production and some 36 hours later the follicle ruptures and the now matured egg is released ('ovulation', say day 14).

The egg(s) that is released is only potentially fertilisable for the next 12 hours.

The cells left behind in the ovary that were lining the follicle from which the egg has been released change to yellow in colour (the corpus luteum). These cells continue to produce further E2 and also progesterone. The progesterone acts on the endometrial lining to alter the quality to one that can nourish an early implanted embryo. This is called the luteal or secretory phase, lasting from day 14 to 28. Unless pregnancy occurs, and the hormone human chorionic gonadotrophin hormone (hCG) starts to be secreted to sustain the life of the corpus luteum beyond its 14-day lifespan, its cells die and hormone secretion stops. Without the sustaining progesterone, the endometrial lining starts to slough off and menstruation occurs. The negative feedback of E2 and progesterone on the hypothalamic-pituitary-axis consequently diminishes, allowing increased production of GnRH, so FSH production increases and the next cycle commences.

The exact trigger mechanism that starts this process at puberty is not fully understood. The process stops when all stimulatable eggs have been used up (potentially 300,000). During the reproductive phase of female life, menstrual cycles usually continue automatically. However, higher centres in the brain (called the supra-tentorial control) via a system called the limbic system may exercise overall overriding control.

The above is not, however, the full story as known today. There are other influences. For instance, pheromones with and without detectable odour have been shown to influence the proliferative phase and LH production. Also, the commencement of the LH surge and consequently the time of oocyte release has been found to alter seasonally. It has been shown that the majority of women ovulate in the morning in spring and in the evening in autumn and winter.

Main causes of ovulatory problems

Physiological causes

Anovulation (absence of ovulation) may be normal, as in pregnancy and usually during lactation (breast feeding) and, of course, after menopause. Pre-puberty the ovaries are not 'switched on' and it is thought the pubescent girl usually needs to reach a weight of at least 45 kg to make this happen and a shift upwards in body fat composition from 16 to 24%.

Any cycle can occasionally be anovulatory. It has been suggested that this happens in 5% at any given time and more often over the age of 40. Ovaries may just stop functioning early if the number of eggs runs out (premature ovarian failure), especially if numbers are low at the start.

Pathological causes

Ovulation may never start, or may stop prematurely, if vital organs or their infrastructure are absent or diseased, or if vital control processes

Figure 10 Some of the main changes that occur during the menstrual cycle (based on 28-day cycle)

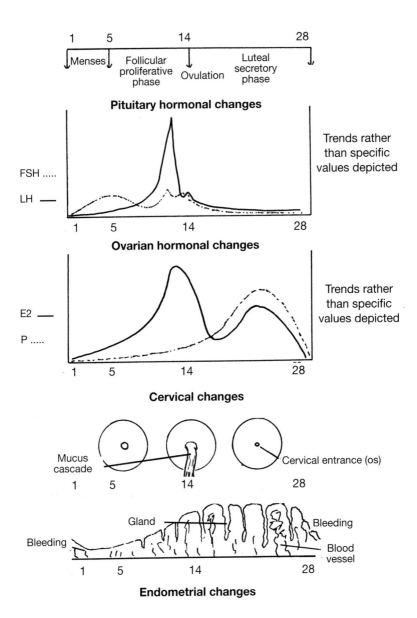

are affected at any level. From the hypothalamic-pituitary-axis to the ovaries, there can be congenital absence or underdevelopment of functioning cells. This may be genetic in origin, such as occurs in Turner's syndrome where one of the X chromosomes is missing. The karyotype is 46X0 instead of 46XX (see chapter 2, page 5) and the ovaries fail to develop. They are described as 'streak gonads' and the females are invariably of small stature. Their ovaries either never work, giving rise to primary amenorrhoea (no periods ever), or more rarely work for a bit and then stop. Secondary amenorrhoea is then the result (periods used to come, now stopped) due to premature menopause. Other possible causes include damage to the blood supply, organ destruction due to tumour formation (with or without hormone secretion), infection, and auto-immune disease and its repair.

Iatrogenic causes

An iatrogenic problem is one caused by a healthcare intervention and includes damage caused by surgical removal of pituitary tumours and ovaries, Sheehan's syndrome is where the pituitary gland is damaged beyond repair, due to inadequately treated severe haemorrhage during or after childbirth. Cancer therapy, in particular radiotherapy of the pelvis, can affect the ovaries. It can destroy 100% of ovarian function if 250-500 rads is given in the pelvic area. Some chemotherapy treatments for cancer, such as alkylating agents, can also cause anovulation by damaging the ovarian cells.

Anovulation after stopping taking the contraceptive pill can also be described as iatrogenic, but the effect is usually temporary.

Toxins

Toxins may cause problems with ovulation. A history of using street drugs and/or smoking is associated with a decrease of one third in female fertility.

The higher centres

The higher centres of the brain (supratentorial control) can halt ovulation via the limbic system, either temporarily or even permanently. This may be the mechanism in stress-related amenorrhoea (absence of periods; see chapter 10, page 164) and contribute to other situations associated with anovulation, such as sudden excessive weight loss, anorexia nervosa (1% of women under 25 years), bulaemia, excessive exercise, and excessive fear of, or desire for, pregnancy.

Other hormonal (endocrine) systems in the body

Any of the other hormone systems in the body, if functioning and secreting abnormally, may impinge on and adversely influence the delicate cycle of ovulation and menstruation (see Figure 12, page 121). A common cause is a tumour in a particular gland that can result in it secreting an excessive amount of its hormones. An example is a tumour of the adrenal gland producing abnormally large quantities of the male hormone testosterone, which causes amenorrhoea as well as hirsutism (excess hair in inappropriate male-type locations).

The most common of these types of tumours are those found in the brain that can lead to excessive prolactin. Prolactin is produced primarily in the pituitary gland under the control of a hypothalamic inhibitory hormone to initiate breast milk production. Overproduction of prolactin by a prolactin-secreting tumour (a prolactinoma) will raise prolactin blood levels and thereby cause anovulation. Excessive stress may also need to be considered as a possible cause as prolactin is a stress hormone (see below and chapter 10, page 164).

Malfunctioning of the thyroid and adrenal glands can also affect ovulation but is more uncommon.

Unclear

Sometimes, the underlying causative endocrine pathway is not entirely clear. This is the case where polycystic ovaries (PCO) are found and the separate but usually linked polycystic ovarian syndrome (PCOs), where androgens (male-type hormones, such as testosterone) and insulin levels may be increased. PCOs is specifically discussed later in this chapter (see page 129).

Luteal phase defect

Luteal phase defect, also known as 'inadequate luteal phase', describes the possibility that while ovulation apparently does occur, the timing of the associated endometrial changes in the uterus is behind the usual pattern thus making the post-ovulatory phase of the cycle and its hormonal output shorter than the normal 14 days (10 days or less).

Some fertility experts consider this to be a recurring phenomenon, possibly causing implantation failure and therefore a significant cause of infertility rather than an isolated chance finding. They link it to a progesterone deficiency. Others deny its existence at all.

Unruptured follicles

Follicles do not always rupture and release an egg, although the corpus luteum may still form. This is called the luteinised unruptured follicle (LUF) syndrome. It is unlikely to be a recurrent happening and the link to infertility is tenuous although cited in IVF literature, particularly as a reason for failing to obtain eggs from follicles of apparently normal size.

Resistant ovary syndrome

Resistant ovary syndrome has been described by some experts as the situation where an ovary with an apparently normal structure that does contain eggs but fails to respond to normal hormonal stimulation. This is very rare and as long-standing secondary amenorrhoea occurs that does not respond to ovulation stimulation, it can be mixed up with premature menopause. Hormone levels, however, tend to be relatively normal unlike premature menopause, which is associated with high FSH and LH and low E2.

Chapter 9

Is ovulation occurring?

History

To determine whether ovulation is likely to be occurring or not, a full menstrual history is necessary. You will be asked about the onset of your periods (menarche) and their quality, such as regularity or otherwise, flow, amount and pain. The link between ovulation and the menstrual cycle can usually give a clear indication of a possible problem. For example, when periods have never started, cycles are abnormally long (oligomenorrhoic for over three months), or stop (amenorrhoic for over six months). This can occur in over 4% of women of reproductive age. This, however, needs to be differentiated from amenorrhoea due to secondary blockage of the outflow tract for menses or to disease or absence of the uterus (chapter 8, pages 72, 74).

Other important questions include past history of disease, drugs, diet, weight fluctuations, voice changes and excessive hair growth (hirsutism) or breast discharge, for how long any symptom or sign has been present and any treatment for it. Any similar ovulatory problems in other family members will also be noted.

Physical examination

A full examination of all systems can be expected with specific emphasis on height and breast development and if there are any lumps or galactorrhoea (milky nipple discharge). Also whether the woman is under or over weight or is hirsute (excessive body hair or body hair in unusual areas).

Basic physiological tests

Having regular menstrual cycles does suggest ovulation is occurring but is not diagnostic of an egg actually being released or of when ovulation occurs. The only definitive proof is actual conception. This is, however, not much use as a method of investigation! Therefore, whether a problem in this area is suspected or not, and to help optimal coital timing, it is customary to institute some way of seeing if ovulation is taking place. Negative findings can then be followed up in depth as necessary.

Basal body temperatures (BBTs) and cervical mucus

Basal body temperatures (BBT) can be charted daily (see Figure 11, page 117) over a period of a few months, with the aim of detecting the sudden drop in level (nadir) that occurs at the time of ovulation and the rise to a plateau that is seen in the luteal phase. BBTs can then be recorded to try to detect problems and monitor treatment. A combination of BBTs and observations of cervical mucus secretions, which become very thin and runny (like egg white) in the peri-ovular phase, can also be used. (This approach is known as Billing's method in natural planning circles.) (See also NaProTechnology, Chapter 10, pages 179-82.)

While used by many, both of these methods are indirect measures as to whether ovulation is occurring and despite strenuous claims to the contrary are likely to be inexact. They are time-consuming and stressful and do not definitively detect ovulation itself, but only the changes elsewhere that take place around that 'more fertile' time.

Home-kit ovulation testing methods

Initially developed for contraception purposes, do-it-yourself (DIY) kits are now available over the counter for home use to detect the peri-ovular phase (see also chapter 5, pages 23-4). Some people use daily urine samples to detect the LH surge and others, oestrogen levels in saliva, which rise towards ovulation increasing salt levels. In the peri-ovular phase, the increased salt becomes visible as crystals under the microscope that is supplied in the kit for this latter test. Both methods claim high accuracy (98-99%) and suggest they can narrow down the phase of 'greatest fertility' to some two to three days. One urine kit quotes a 6% pregnancy rate.

These methods suffer from the same problems as temperature charts and are best applicable where ovulatory cycles are regular and coital or AI timing (see chapter 11, page 198) is wanted. They are not sufficiently accurate at present to use where ovulation is irregular or where ovulation is being induced in anovulation situations.

Hormone assays

A satisfactorily high progesterone level measured in the mid-luteal phase (day 20-24) in a regular 28-day cycle does suggest that ovulation has occurred. It does not, however, confirm that an egg has been released, or when this has occurred. A guarantee that the next cycle will be the same cannot be made. To test each cycle is generally impractical. This is the Achilles heel of all ovulation function tests.

Figure 11 Diagrams of typical basal body temperature (BBT) charts

Chart indicating ovulation

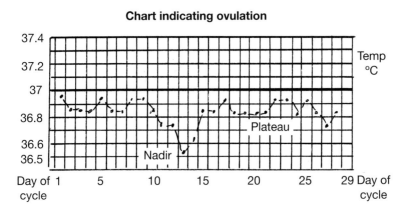

Chart indicating no ovulation

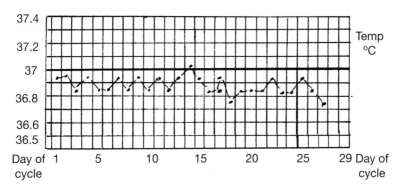

Ovarian ultrasound (US) scans

Abdominal or vaginal ultrasound tracking can be used to follow the growth of a follicle (the fluid-filled sac containing the egg) in the ovary serially through to its disappearance at ovulation. This is the most exact method at present available, especially when performed trans-vaginally (see Figure 17, page 220). It is very useful as it is possible to look at the site, size and appearance of the ovaries in a relatively non-invasive way and to monitor ovulation induction therapy. However, utilising it serially solely as a diagnostic agent is impractical and, as with any test aimed at detecting ovulation on a one-cycle basis, offers no guarantee that the same thing is going to happen in the next cycle.

Laparoscopy

At operation it is possible to see by chance that ovulation is about to happen or has recently occurred. Scars on the ovaries formed by healing of the site of egg release from the ripe follicle may also show that it has in the past. Obviously this is impractical as a monitoring device.

Uterine curettage

Histological examination of the endometrium was often used in the past to 'date' changes in the cells that alter appearance at different times of the cycle, in order to give information on ovulation and possible problems with the cycle. It is invasive and could disturb a very early pregnancy.

Investigating causes of ovarian dysfunction

Hormone assays – the hormone profile

Even if a woman's menstrual cycle history is normal and she seems to be ovulating, because the mechanism of menstrual cycle control is hormonal, when ovulation problems are suspected it is logical to investigate the specific hormones involved (see Figures 10 and 12, pages 111 and 121) as the likely cause of the trouble. Because ovulation is a key to fertility, a 'hormone profile', is one of the basic initial investigations in the overall fertility profile. The results of such tests can also provide a pointer to whether treatment may be possible and what might be most suitable.

FSH, LH and E2 are often measured in the menstrual phase (days 3-5) and again, together with progesterone, in the mid-luteal phase (days 20-24). It is not customary to try to search for the LH surge. Prolactin levels are also often routinely tested using the same blood samples or if galactorrhoea is present and, if a problem is suspected clinically, thyroid function tests will be carried out. If the woman is inappropriately hairy (hirsute) or is suspected of having polycystic ovarian syndrome, male hormones (androgens) such as testosterone are also measured, and sometimes insulin (see later in this chapter, page 130).

I have not quoted specific hormone levels here, even from my own clinic, as these can vary between laboratories due to different methodologies; each laboratory should be able to supply what the normal ranges are for their specific approach. However, in basic terms, low FSH, LH and E2 suggests under-functioning of the hypothalamic-pituitary axis. This is potentially treatable by stimulation with drugs (the so-called fertility drugs). High FSH and LH in the presence of low E2 suggests ovarian failure, which is not treatable. A raised prolactin level may indicate a benign pituitary tumour; this will be followed up by skull MRI (magnetic resonance imaging) or similar. Stress may also raise prolactin levels, but not usually as high (see pages 167-8).

Hormone stimulation tests

Hormone stimulation tests can be used to test hormonal function further. The one most used by gynaecologists at present seems to be the clomiphene challenge test. This is used to assess the woman's ovarian reserve, which can be in doubt if routine day-3 FSH levels, controlled for age, are slightly higher than the normal range (near or above 15 IU/litre). If clomiphene citrate is then given for five days (clomid challenge test) and the FSH result on day 10, compared with baseline on day 3, is significantly raised, this indicates the ovarian reserve (number of eggs still present in the ovary) may be low and there is likely to be a poor response to ovarian stimulation. This is particularly important in ovarian stimulation for IVF. Other tests can also be employed in this situation (see page 122 and chapter 11, page 214).

Chromosome tests

Primary or long-term secondary amenorrhoea suggests the possibility of premature ovarian failure. This may be genetic in origin. Chromosome analysis can be performed to help diagnose the underlying cause (see Turner's syndrome as discussed above, page 112) if the woman's history or the findings of physical examination suggest the need.

Main treatments

General diseases of hormonal origin are often investigated and treated by endocrine physicians. Their aid may still be sought by the infertility clinic when a specific endocrine organ dysfunction is found that could have implications for general health. However, as far as the menstrual cycle and ovulation abnormalities are concerned, when the problem is one of trying to conceive, it is generally thought preferable nowadays for women to be investigated and treated by the gynaecologist in charge of their fertility problem. When the situation is complex or requires gonadotrophin therapy, someone with specific gynaecological-endocrinological training needs to be involved; this should be available in any tertiary care unit. He/she will also be likely to be more used than an endocrine physician to carrying out any appropriate intimate female examinations, have the wherewithal to monitor therapy on site, and have the training and experience to deal with any early pregnancies that may occur.

None possible

In a number of situations it will be found that direct treatment cannot be offered. This includes in-born defects such as testicular feminisation (the woman has male XY chromosomes and gonads but a female external appearance) and situations where ovaries are congenitally absent. These can appear as streak ovaries (Turner's X0 syndrome) where ovarian function never starts, or fails prematurely (45XX, 46X0). Ovarian function may also fail due to disease such as some forms of cancer or its

Figure 12 Algorithm of the menstrual cycle hormonal control

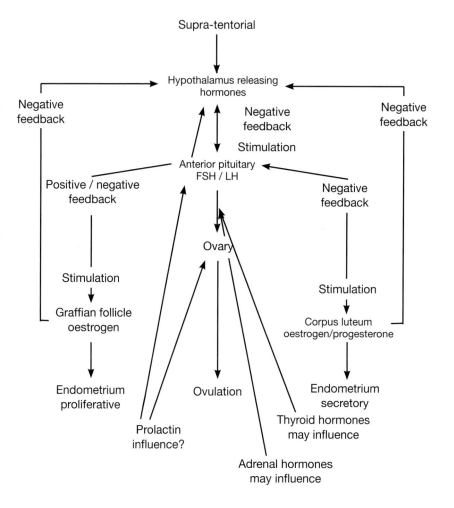

treatment by chemotherapy or radiation. However, the problem is often 'idiopathic' (unknown cause).

In resistant ovary syndrome, hormone levels appear normal but the ovaries seem incapable of responding to the hormones produced. Gonadotrophin treatment has been tried almost to no avail. In rare circumstances, ovulation may re-start spontaneously.

In all cases of true ovarian failure, FSH and LH levels will be found to be very high and E2 low (menopausal levels). This signals that using ovarian stimulating drugs will not work. Then close guidance and expert counselling are essential. In some circumstances, hormone replacement therapy (HRT) may be needed. The possibility of using donor eggs may also be worth considering at this point (see page 213).

If ovarian stimulation is possible...

This section excludes the specifics of stimulating the ovaries in the presence of PCOs as this is dealt with in depth below (pages 129-35).

General lifestyle

Good general lifestyle is as important as a good diet. If the woman is morbidly obese this will need to be addressed both from a general health viewpoint and to optimise ovarian function and the likelihood of pregnancy occurring. Gradual weight reduction may help to restart ovulation naturally and also give ovarian stimulation a better chance of working. However, the ability of the ovaries to respond decreases as age increases, particularly over 35 years of age. Ovarian reserve lessens and then, having no apparent chance of success, treatment may become inadvisable.

Although possibly not always an exact predictor as mentioned above (page 119), higher than normal basal FSH and LH levels on day 3 of the cycle can indicate that the woman has a poor ovarian reserve (fewer available eggs to be stimulated). A clomiphene challenge test may confirm it. Newer tests, such as counting of early ('antral') follicles by ultrasound, or determining blood levels of inhibin B, or, most lately, of anti-Mullerian hormone (AMH), may yet prove to be better markers.

If the reproductive system is intact, levels of FSH and LH are low to normal, and there is a real indication that it will be worthwhile without risking the woman's health untowardly, an attempt at stimulating the ovaries using 'fertility drugs' can always be explored with the couple.

Anti-oestrogen drugs

The most frequent method of stimulating ovarian function is the use of what is classified as the anti-oestrogen group of drugs, particularly clomiphene citrate (CC). Tamoxifen citrate is also used, but less frequently. CC is given by mouth, starting with 50-100 milligrams (max 200 milligrams) daily for four to five days frequently from day 2-3 of the cycle for up to six months.

Follicle tracking of the response by ultrasound is not always used even though multiple pregnancy is quite common (10% plus). Some couples prefer to await the clinical response; others use basal body temperatures.

Anti-oestrogens seem to influence the negative E2 pituitary feedback loop (see Figure 12, page 121) by blocking the pituitary oestrogen reception cells as FSH and LH levels rise. This enables the pituitary output of FSH to continue at a higher level.

The indications for CC treatment are (1) anovulation with low FSH and LH levels but reasonable E2 levels, and (2) the presence of polycystic ovarian syndrome (see below). However, anti-oestrogens are also often sadly misused in other infertility situations. They are prescribed to 'ensure ovulation is really working'. This includes especially unexplained infertility (chapter 10, pages 173-82). Pregnancy rates based on meta-analysis of a wide range of studies give an incidence of some 5.6% only compared with over 40% where genuinely indicated. In addition, they are sometimes given for far too long (over six months) when genuinely indicated, even when it is obvious that even the maximum dosage is not working.

Side effects may include headaches, hot flushes, mood swings, visual disturbance and abdominal discomfort. Cervical mucus can become scanty and the endometrium remain thin. The likelihood of multiple pregnancy (especially twins), ectopic pregnancy and hyperstimulation is increased, though the latter two remain rare.

Combined and concomitant therapies

Sometimes used in combination with the anti-oestrogens are such treatments as hCG (human chorionic gonadotrophin) injections mid-cycle to simulate an LH surge that will time ovulation (see also chapter 11, page 199) or where a luteal phase defect is suggested. Oestrogens can be given in the peri-ovular phase if cervical mucus seems to be diminished. Prescribing an aromatase-inhibitor class of drug plus CC is a new innovation (see PCOs section below in which other combinations with CC, including oral diabetic agents and steroids, are also discussed).

With research collaborators I have investigated very mild hyperprolactinaemia (slightly raised prolactin blood levels) as a possible stress response (stress spikes) to the infertility situation, and found a combination of clomiphene and the dopamine agonist drug called bromocriptine to be better than placebo in achieving pregnancies. Additionally, we found that non-medical relaxation therapy certainly lowered prolactin levels and some of the women concerned did conceive (see chapter 10, pages 170 and 171-2, and chapter 12, page 248).

Gonadotrophin treatment

Where FSH and LH levels are extremely low or anti-oestrogens fail to stimulate ovulation, at that stage and only at that stage (apart from with ART see chapter 11, pages 207, 217) should the gonadotophin (FSH/LH) drugs be used, and even then, only in a specialised clinic setting with full direct monitoring facilities. For safety's sake, a course of treatment should be embarked on only if suitably experienced and trained staff are available, as should be the case in a tertiary care centre.

The idea behind the treatment is to stimulate the ovaries, as occurs naturally, but with externally given gonadotrophins because the body itself has failed in its own FSH/LH gonadotrophin production. These days this family of drugs is either obtained by extraction/purification of FSH and LH from human menopausal urine (u) or is artificially made (recombinant, 'r'). The end result can be either to use purified uFSH or rFSH, pure rLH or a mixture of different ratios of urinary-extracted to recombinant FSH and LH. The LH in the urinary product is supplemented with hCG to make it more standardised in its batch to batch dosage. Human chorionic gonadotrophin (hCG) is itself extracted from pregnant women's urine. It is also used when the other gonadotrophins are used to simulate the LH surge pre-ovulation as it acts in the body pre-ovulation just like LH – that is, it matures the egg and acts as an LH surge.

FSH or FSH/LH is given by daily injections, administered carefully, often starting in the non-IVF situation with very low dosages and 'stepping up' in a dose-response manner, always monitoring the effect closely with ultrasound plus perhaps E2 assays. When follicular development is sufficient (18-20 mm size on ultrasound) a single dose of hCG (usually 5000 IU) or more rarely rLH is then injected to finalise ovum (egg) development and cause ovulation to occur.

The response to this therapy is difficult to predict and control. It may differ even from one cycle to the next in the same patient. Because of this, especially in IVF (chapter 11, page 216), to try to make it more predictable, gonadotrophin treatment may also be combined with the use of what are called GnRH agonists or antagonists. Make sure you receive pre-treatment counselling as to what is involved and possible side-effects as this is essential.

Multiple pregnancy (up to 40%) and the life-threatening side effects of ovarian hyperstimulation syndrome (OHSS, 1-2%) are always possible, although lessened in experienced hands and with good monitoring. If OHSS occurs, it is often mild and resolves with time, though pregnancy will prolong it. However, there is always the potential for hospitalisation, severe illness, organ function loss and even death. To aid safety and efficacy, strict protocols when monitoring with ultrasound and also possibly blood oestradiol (E2) levels need to be in place. Used purely in this clinical (non-IVF) context, signs of over-stimulation (3+ follicles developing) will necessitate immediate discontinuation.

GnRH

Where the hypothalamus itself is not functioning and the relevant stimulatory hormones therefore not being produced, a gonadotrophin releasing hormone (GnRH) can be used, administered in a 'pulsatile fixed frequency' manner via a pump and needle to simulate hypothalamic function. The woman wears the pump continuously with the needle placed subcutaneously. The drug is given over a period of a few weeks to try to stimulate the pituitary itself to work, produce FSH and LH and in turn thus stimulate ovarian function (see earlier, page 108).

Dopamine agonists

Where prolactin levels are significantly raised and there is no ovulation, one of the group of drugs known as dopamine agonists (commonly bromocriptine, daily, or cabergoline, weekly) can be prescribed alone. Nausea is a common side effect, but the drugs do lower the prolactin level very efficiently, allowing the ovaries to recommence their ordinary function.

When the cause of the hyperprolactinaemia is a tumour (prolactinoma) in the pituitary region, neurosurgery may need to be considered on rare occasions first. The drugs also importantly stop galactorrhoea, shrink prolactinomas and bromocriptine can be continued during a pregnancy to counteract the natural enlargement that occurs in the pituitary region of the brain during this time; this is necessary because if there is already some enlargement even further enlargement can temporarily affect the woman's sight owing to proximity to the optic nerve.

IVF

As with all other infertility factors, IVF is the final port of call for treatable anovulation. It may even need to be considered the primary approach to treatment if there are other factors in addition to anovulation needing IVF, or if gonadotrophin treatment alone is impractical or likely to be dangerous.

Prognosis for fertility

The prognoses given in this next section exclude cases where the treatment has been given because of PCOs (polycystic ovarian syndrome) as this is discussed separately on pages 129-35).

General

While it may be possible to calculate percentages of cycles where ovulation has been stimulated and pregnancy achieved per a single ovulation cycle, in all ovarian stimulation situations other than IVF, where per cycle calculations are the norm (see chapter 11, page 238-9), it is customary to refer to the percentage of women who get pregnant over a fixed period of time or a specific number of cycles undergone (per six months or six cycles is often chosen).

As with all infertility treatment, the woman's age enters the equation as it can alter expected outcome and the potential for side effects. Many women can be helped to ovulate but not all will conceive. For those who do, it is interesting to note that a number will conceive again spontaneously within the next two to three years, as a result of either a placebo effect or the pregnancy restoring normality to the cyclic hormonal control.

Treatment not possible

If no treatment is possible, the prognosis is nil unless donor eggs are used with IVF. The prognosis will then be commensurate with the age of the donor, the number and quality of eggs available to inseminate and the woman's health (see pages 122 and 237).

Ovulation stimulation with drugs is possible

Where the indications are medically valid and not just a 'to be sure to be sure' situation, all the therapies discussed above (anti-oestrogen or gonadotrophin) when used alone may be expected to stimulate ovulation successfully in 80% of women and have an up to 60-65% cumulative pregnancy rate over a six-month course of treatment. The majority of successes with both gonadotrophin and anti-oestrogen therapy occur in the first three months. Prognosis for success is poor after six months' continuous treatment. Miscarriage rates are usually within the normally expected range (around 20%) but ectopic rates appear higher.

A combination of clomiphene and bromocriptine has been found to be similarly effective (including in women with polycystic ovarian syndrome) and controlled studies by myself and others have shown this to be statistically significantly better than placebo (64% compared with 21%), but only where stress spikes of prolactin have been found. Some other scientifically designed placebo-controlled studies on oral products for inducing ovulation, such as CC with or without hCG, and bromocriptine alone, have also been performed by the author and others. However, where there is no proper indication for ovulation induction, all studies have shown that efficacy drops over the 6-12 month administration period to an equivalent of the maximum placebo response (see chapter 5, page 26-7) – that is, some 20-30%. This is a very important factor to bear in mind (see also chapter 10, Unexplained infertility prognosis, pages 175-82). It needs to be weighed against potential side effects from these powerful oral treatments if the indications are not clear. These may include the usual nausea, vomiting, allergies, bowel upsets, and stress, together with disappointment at failure due to unrealistic expectations.

As well as these, there are also the two major complications to consider, both of which are dose-related and unpredictable. The first is multiple pregnancy; clomiphene citrate gives a twinning incidence of some 10%+ and occasionally triplets. Ovarian hyperstimulation syndrome (OHSS) is the second, as I have already described. Like multiple pregnancies (up to 40%) it is more common with gonadotrophin therapy (1-2%), but can occur very rarely even with anti-oestrogens like clomiphene citrate. In addition, an association has been suggested between prolonged usage of these drugs and cancer. At present there is little evidence to support this when they have been used for under 12 months at the lowest possible effective dosages.

GnRH

With this rarely used but effective therapy, side effects are minimal, with multiple births and hyperstimulation rarely occurring. However, wearing a noisy pump to send drugs into the body at constant intervals over some weeks can be very tiring.

POLYCYSTIC OVARIAN SYNDROME (PCOS)

General

PCOs is the most commonly cited single cause of ovulation problems. The prevalence in the general population in women of reproductive age is estimated at 6-7% (1:15). But in infertile women, where an ovulation factor is present, some 75% will be found to have PCOs. As such, the condition deserves a special section to itself in this chapter.

What is PCOs?

PCOs cannot be diagnosed without first eliminating other problems such as thyroid disease, adrenal hyperplasia, hyperprolactinaemia, male hormone secreting tumours in the ovary and Cushing's disease (over-secretion of the steroid cortisol). It is a metabolic condition, commonly associated with insulin resistance, as occurs with diabetes mellitus. It has typical clinical, biochemical and ovarian features on ultrasound. However, even in the presence of a strong family or typical personal history, over the years, the diagnosis of PCOs has become so confused, especially in terms of hormonal parameters, that joint meetings of the American Society for Reproductive Medicine (ASRM) and its European counterpart (ESHRE) have been held to discuss how best to make the diagnosis more definitive.

These expert groups stated (Rotterdam, 2003, published in *Human Reproduction* 2004; 19(1): 41-47) that a diagnosis of PCOs can be sustained only in the presence of at least two of three clinical signs: oligo/anovulation (infrequent/absence of ovulation), clinical and/ or biological signs of hyperandrogenism (acne, hirsutism, deepening voice, high male hormone levels), and ultrasound evidence of polycystic ovaries (enlarged, with many small cysts).

Controversy, however, continues and recently a majority report of the Androgen Excess and PCOS Society Multinational Task Force (in *Fertility and Sterility* 2009; 91(2): 456-488) published their criteria for diagnosis of the syndrome. These require the presence of: hyperandrogrenism (clinical and/or biochemical), ovarian dysfunction (oligo/anovulation with or without polycystic ovaries), and exclusion of related disorders. A minority of Task Force members felt hyperandrogenism did not need to be present in some forms of PCOs. All expected further evolution of the definition with time.

Clinical suspicions

Fifty to sixty per cent of women with PCOs are overweight, although some 5% are lean. Periods are infrequent ('oligomenorrhic' – a cycle of three to six months in length) or amenorrhoic (no periods for over six months). Oligomenorrhoea occurs in 76% and many are hyperandrogenic-looking, with acne, hirsutism (excessive hairiness) or alopecia (loss of head hair).

Hormone, ultrasound and ovarian structural changes

In the basic hormone profile, the ratio of LH to FSH will more often than not be abnormal (more than 3:1 compared with the normal ratio of approximately 1:1). Levels of free testosterone (the male hormone) may be raised mildly but not always. Hyperinsulinism due to excessive insulin resistance may be detected (30-40%). On vaginal examination or at laparoscopy, the doctor may find the ovaries appear enlarged and hard. On ultrasound scan or seen directly at operation, the PCO ovary is typically enlarged (10 cm^3) with a rosette of small follicles (12+ in number, like rosary beads, less than 10 mm in diameter) around the periphery. However, while this can be linked to PCOs and anovulation, such appearances may also be seen in up to 25% of normal women.

Ovarian biopsy (taking a tiny piece of the ovary for viewing under a microscope) shows a thickened ovarian capsule (skin). This was first described in the 1930s by Stein and Leventhal who gave the syndrome its alternative name, still sometimes used for severe cases.

Treatment of PCOs in infertility

Primary approach

The primary approach to treatment is symptom orientated, aimed at trying to correct first anovulation, menstrual irregularities and skin manifestations. Controlled supervised weight loss back towards the normal body mass index (BMI: see chapter 4, page 16) for the woman's height, where necessary, can by itself restore ovulation and fertility in up to 90%. It is important that where indicated this is tried first and continued even if additional therapy is then needed.

Where pregnancy is then achieved, screening for gestational diabetes before 20 weeks' gestation is advisable.

Ovarian stimulation

If a woman with PCOs wants to conceive, anti-oestrogen therapy (especially clomiphene citrate) is principally used. Indeed, this is regarded after counselling and weight management as the first choice active management by an ESHRE/ASRM concensus group who met in Thessaloniki in 2007 (published in *Human Reproduction* 2008; 23(3): 462-477).

As I said earlier in this chapter, up to 80% of patients will respond, the other 20% being clomiphene resistant (fail to ovulate despite increasing dosages). Some 40-65% may conceive within six months.

In PCOs patients with poor insulin tolerance, oral insulin sensitising agents have also been prescribed. Biguanide/metformin hydrochloride, which is used in type 2 diabetes, has been reported to enhance clomiphene efficacy, especially when there is clomiphene resistance, and can also have a positive effect on insulin resistance if this is also a problem. However, except in PCOs patients of normal weight, placebo-controlled studies of the mixture (also including metformin plus gonadotrophin pre-IVF) have been less enthusiastic. Additionally, when used alone in this situation, metformin results have also been reported as poor and no better than with the placebo. Its continuation on into pregnancy is not at present recommended.

The addition of bromocriptine may enhance results, but only where stress spikes of prolactin have been found. If hyperandrogenism and hirsutism are present, the addition of the steroid dexamethasone may enhance the response to clomiphene citrate.

Gonadotrophins can also be used when clomiphene fails to stimulate ovulation, but these must only be used with extreme care and with very close direct monitoring by ultrasound, plus or minus oestradiol blood levels, starting with the lowest of doses. PCOs patients are very susceptible to hyperstimulation. Large numbers of follicles can sometimes form. If treatment is continued, multiple pregnancies and OHSS are then the likely outcomes (see above and chapter 11, page 234). With care, pregnancy rates of around 40% can be expected, but miscarriage rates are higher than the normal estimate of some 15-20%, epecially if the woman is still obese with a high BMI (see chapter 4, page 16).

Not yet indicated officially for conditions other than breast cancer, aromatase inhibitors such as letrozole and anastrozole, which also inhibit the formation of oestradiol (E2), have recently been used with some success by themselves early in the cycle in PCOs women after clomiphene treatment had failed (regularly ovulating on treatment but no pregnancy after six to nine months), or in combination with clomiphene and also gonadotrophins. Aromatase inhibitors plus gonadotrophins allow lower dosages of gonadotrophins to be used. A non-randomised but controlled study of IUI (intra-uterine insemination) plus gonadotrophin plus an aromatase inhibitor in women with PCOs has shown specifically significantly lower cycle cancellations and higher pregnancy rates than IUI plus gonadotrophin alone (26.5% compared with 18.5%).

Operative treatment

Women with PCOs used to have wedge resection of the ovaries performed at laparotomy to reduce ovarian volume. A sizeable slice was removed from each and the ovaries then reconstituted (sewn up again). This procedure has been supplanted by laparoscopic ovarian diathermy of the rosette of cysts by electrocautery or laser (ovarian drilling). Up to 60% of women who have had these latter treatments have found that while insulin sensitivity was unaltered, androgen (male hormone) levels fell quickly and they started ovulating, especially those with a normal BMI. The reason why this happens is not fully known but the surgery may have destroyed sufficient androgen-producing tissue to change the environment to one that promoted oestrogen production. The problem with such surgery on the ovaries is the potential for adhesions to form, affecting the ovum pick-up mechanism (see Figure 7, page 80). Unlike with drug therapy, this may be irreversible so such procedures should be carefully planned after full discussions have taken place.

Long-term prognosis

Preventative strategies are needed, particularly if the woman is obese. There are other health implications as well as infertility. Often, but not always, glucose tolerance can be affected and by the age of 40 a minimum of some 10-20% women will develop type 2 diabetes. The incidence of sleep apnoea (respiratation stops transiently during sleep) is increased, and there may be an increased risk of cardiovascular problems later on, but definitive evidence is not yet available. However, many obese PCOs women share features of the 'metabolic syndrome' (alias 'insulin resistance syndrome'). This is a collection of medical disorders including obesity, hypertension, abnormally high blood triglycerides and insulin resistance. Such patients have an increasing risk of developing cardiovascular problems and diabetes.

Long-term hyperoestrogenism without progesterone, as occurs in chronic oligomenorrhoea, may give rise to endometrial overgrowth (hyperplasia) and possibly endometrial cancer. For this reason, if a woman with PCOs is not trying to conceive, it may be good practice to take progesterone supplements at intervals to produce withdrawal bleeds.

The effects of high androgen levels on skin quality and hair growth (excessive) can affect general wellbeing and be difficult to cope with. A combination of various cosmetic measures is often used. Anti-androgens can help but this is of no use to a woman desperately wanting to conceive as pregnancy needs to be avoided when on such therapy.

Personal Comment

Ovarian malfunctions are thought to be common but are often intermittent and may self correct. Charting physiological symptoms and signs over months is unreliable and, in my experience, can be stressful for patients, especially if used to try to time coitus or when time is of the essence due to increasing age and length of infertility. Reasonably reliable diagnostic agents are available, but to use these in each cycle may be impractical. Beware that findings in one cycle may not be the same in the next. Therefore aiming maximum coital efforts at what you think is the most fertile time can be counter productive. It is far better to do it 'when you fancy' any time through the cycle, provided of course that you fancy it often enough (every two to three days or so), if possible as part of proper 'love making sessions'. Ovulation stimulation agents are much prescribed, alone and in conjunction with other drugs where symptoms or signs suggest a possible benefit. However, I feel strongly that there must be a valid indication for their use and proper monitoring facilities. Pressure to use 'fertility drug' treatment comes from all sides, even when there are no indications. This situation is unlikely to change in the near future, until ignorance regarding true efficacy and the potential for serious side effects is truly out in the open for all potential recipients and prescribers to see.

Anti-oestrogens are in particular greatly misused; empiric (not based on evidence) prescribing 'to be sure to be sure' that ovulation is occurring when it is already likely to be doing so naturally, is sadly very common. In this, all of us practising in the field of infertility are likely to have been guilty at some stage. However, even worse in my opinion is the fact that anti-oestrogens are often used without any tests to indicate whether they may be needed and before referral to an infertility clinic where they can be properly monitored. Where the woman is likely to be ovulating already, scientific evidence reported by myself and others shows anti-oestrogens to be no better than placebo at the best, but with the added danger of side effects.

The use of gonadotrophins can be very effective and they certainly have a place, but it is important to recognise that they are potentially dangerous and should only be used in experienced hands with proper in-house monitoring facilities.

The diagnosis of PCOs is still controversial and almost invariably involves discussion and advice on weight. I acknowledge that this is a delicate and sensitive issue and that we live in an increasingly PC world where terms like 'fat' and 'morbid obesity' are frowned upon, but sometimes I find a lack of realism necessitates 'calling a spade a spade'. To avoid discussing the situation from early on simply because of this sensitivity is a mistake; it is definitely beneficial through frank discussion to get a person(s) to acknowledge there is a problem and try to change. The subject may therefore need to be introduced whether the overweight person likes it or not. If you are in this situation this should not be an occasion for falling out with the staff managing your case; they will be raising weight as an issue only with your best interests at heart.

Chapter 10

Issues affecting both partners

MYTH

It is unusual to find problems in both partners.

As I said at the start of the book, the likelihood of having a child depends on the interaction between the fertility potentials of both partners. This chapter examines how this interaction can be investigated. In particular, I explore the cervical factor – what to do when coitus does not or cannot occur, the role stress may play in the whole process and what the options are when no explanation for infertility can be found. In the final section, I look at 'recurrent miscarriage', where again both partners need to be considered together.

SECTION I: THE CERVICAL FACTOR AND THE POST-COITAL TEST

Why is the cervical region important?

Testing the cervix, or neck of the womb - that is, the entrance to the body of the uterus (see Figures 1 and 3, pages 5 and 32) - is the first, and indeed the only, practical way of looking at how the couple interact inside the woman's body. It has the potential to reveal valuable information on the adequacy or otherwise of penetrative intercourse as well as problems with semen, and with the ovulation cycle and its control in the woman.

It is important to note that not all authorities on infertility see the value in testing specifically and formally for problems in this region. A positive post-coital test (PCT) and the number of sperm seen in one do not correlate with the chances of pregnancy. Therefore, too much should not be read into positive or negative post-coital test results. There is, in particular, doubt as to the existence of a specific barrier to conception operating in the cervix area, the so-called immunologically based 'cervical factor' (see below). However, despite these caveats, valuable information towards building the overall fertility profile in other areas and discovering hidden psycho-sexual or vaginal examination phobias can still be gleaned by testing this region. It is my opinion, therefore, that it is still appropriate to consider the cervical area as one of the four specific separate regions to be investigated in building the basic fertility profile of an infertile couple.

How the cervical region is investigated

The post-coital test (PCT)

The PCT is the key investigation. This is one of the oldest tests devised in infertility (Sims, 1866). It is performed, if possible, in the peri-ovulatory (around the time of ovulation) phase of the menstrual cycle – that is, in the majority of women around 12 to 14 days after the start of her period. The couple needs to have had unprotected intercourse ideally some eight hours before the scheduled time for the test. A vaginal speculum (see Figure 2, page 30) is used so that the cervix can be visualised and a specimen of cervical mucus taken from the cervical canal (neck of the womb) for further examination.

The quality of the mucus is first evaluated in terms of its quantity, colour and stretchability ('spinnbarkheit'). (Peri-ovular cervical mucus should be like runny egg white.) The mucus specimen is then put on a glass slide and viewed immediately under a microscope at high magnification (x 40). The aim is to see whether sperm are present and to estimate how many can be seen within each field of view at this magnification, their quality and their movement.

Interpretation of the results is controversial. A number of scoring systems have been suggested. The actual number of motile (moving forward purposefully) sperm seen does not define the chances of being able to achieve a pregnancy, but if there are no sperm or only immotile sperm the test result is considered to be negative.

Both positive and negative results should be compared with the data from the spermiogram (see chapter 7, page 49) and from tests of ovulation (chapter 9). The vast majority should agree, but, where correlation is poor or repeat tests are continually negative when coitus is definitely taking place, further in-depth investigation in the area may be needed to try to discover the cause. However, too many repeat PCTs may give rise to stress and, possibly, promote psycho-sexual difficulties (page 154).

Other follow-up cervical region tests when the PCT is negative for no apparent reason

The majority of other tests are based on observing sperm-cervical-mucus interaction without prior intercourse. In the most commonly used form, a drop of semen is placed next to some cervical mucus. The junction between the two is observed under a microscope for a timed interval (maybe 10 minutes) for the ability and distance of the sperm to penetrate the mucus. This is called either a sperm hostility, sperm invasion or sperm penetration test. A number of well-recognised authorities have suggested over many years that poor penetration of 'good quality mucus' by normally motile sperm or seeing violent shaking of the sperm and their eventually dying as they touch the mucus and try to penetrate into it suggests the possible presence of anti-sperm antibody/antigen reaction taking place and a 'cervical factor'. (See also Semen analysis in chapter 7, Male Factor Infertility, page 49-51).

Causes of abnormal PCTs

Causes of PCT abnormalities in this area may be divided into five. Two of these reflect problems in other regions – the male and female genital tract and ovulation. Psycho-sexual difficulties, iatrogenic causes and the so-called 'cervical factor' itself are the others.

Male problems

A negative PCT can be due to poor quality semen. On the other hand, it could be due to an inability to deposit semen appropriately due to a penile anatomical abnormality (see chapter 7, page 48).

Female problems

On the female side, there may be an anatomical defect in the vagina (most commonly a septum) stopping proper deposition of sperm. However, poor quality mucus (dysmucorrhoea) is the most usual reason. The cause of this may be physiological. If the woman is not in fact ovulating the test will not have been performed in the peri-ovular phase. Alternatively, mucus quality may have been damaged by infection in the cervix (cervicitis), or be scantily produced as a side effect of cervical operations or anti-oestrogen ovarian stimulation treatment with clomiphene citrate (see chapter 9, page 123). However, some experts have also suggested a deficit of oestrogen (the hormone that promotes cervical mucus production (see Figure 10, page 111)) may occur even in an ovulatory menstrual cycle.

Psycho-sexual problems in both man and woman

The PCT can confirm whether satisfactory coitus is taking place or not. Unlikely as it may seem today, the couple may not understand what adequate coitus is. Alternatively, they may be too embarrassed to acknowledge to the tester until the PCT test fails that there is a psycho-sexual problem. This may be the only way such a problem is uncovered if a couple are unwilling to come up front about it or do not themselves suspect such a problem exists (see page 151).

The male may have problems with penetration or ejaculation. The female may have 'vaginismus'. This may be the underlying cause of infertility or be a one-off, brought about by the stress of having to have intercourse to order. Fear of passing a speculum is also found but more rarely than fear of penile penetration (see page 160).

Iatrogenic causes

The term 'iatrogenic' is used in relation to the fertility profile when the fault lies with the doctor/clinic in failing to obtain an appropriate specimen, in not organising the test conditions properly or giving the couple inadequate instructions resulting in no coitus or intercourse at the wrong time in the cycle. Also covered by this heading would be ordering tests in the known presence of vaginal medication or failing to instruct about the advisability of using vaginal lubricants as some may affect sperm motility, or stopping douching afterwards.

'True Cervical Factor'?

For many years it has been suggested that a problem detected initially through abnormal PCT and invasion test results, possibly immunological in origin, acting in the cervical region, was a cause of infertility. In some way it was felt the sperm (antigen) were being stopped from penetrating the cervical mucus and were instead being killed-off by the woman's antibodies.

The woman was thought to be the person responsible and tests for 'sperm antibodies' concentrated upon her. These included additional blood tests looking for what were termed 'circulating sperm antibodies'. With these the 'true cervical factor' was estimated as the cause of infertility in some 3% of all cases. However, it is true to say that, following considerable doubt being cast upon the scientific veracity of such tests, nowadays, despite conflicting evidence as to whether such a cause exists at all, what is still termed a possible immunological sperm-antibody factor is now more usually sought by testing the semen for sperm antibodies (MAR and immunobead tests: see chapter 7, pages 49-50) than by looking for it in the female.

As far as the 'cervical factor itself is concerned, today for most workers in the field there is no such a thing as female sperm allergy. The term and concept are historical. They do not test the woman for it or offer treatment to her. However, semen is now routinely tested for the presence of 'sperm antibodies' and where results are positive, washing is used to try to remove them from the sample prior to IUI or IVF/ICSI. But is this not just a different approach to the same old entity? It was termed the 'cervical factor' in error originally because of its known site as the first contact between sperm and the woman.

Therapeutic solutions

Specific male, female or psycho-sexual problems

Any of these problems that are first revealed by a negative post-coital test should be investigated further as per cause (see relevant chapters in the book). Cervical mucus quality may be improved by using low-dose oestrogen tablets given orally for approximately seven days around the anticipated time of ovulation, but there is a possibility of this interfering with ovulation or its timing.

Iatrogenic problems

It is down to the clinic/health professionals to provide clear written and spoken pre-test instructions. If there is anything you do not understand, check this out and seek reassurance as necessary as this is one of the most intimate of investigations that can ever be suggested to you.

The 'cervical factor'

As explained above, the 'cervical factor' was thought in the past to be linked to the presence of sperm antibodies in the female, which reacted against the sperm antigen and killed them off inside her when they came in contact with her cervical region. Diagnosis and treatment concentrated on her. Avoiding coitus or using condoms for some months was suggested to try to lower 'sperm antibody allergy' levels. In the male, steroids in high dosage were prescribed. These approaches were problematic and together with the tests used have now been confined to the history books.

Today investigation of 'sperm antibodies' and their treatment focuses almost exclusively on the semen; the MAR and immunobead tests look for the presence or otherwise of antibodies in semen in sufficient quantities (MAR results are considered to be positive in a concentration over 80%, the immunobead less than 50%).

As a cause of infertility this is, however, still considered unproven. It should be understood that any treatment offered on the basis of such a diagnosis is empiric (not based on scientific research). Treatment is, however, still suggested by many and usually involves attempting to wash the antibodies that have been detected off the sperm. IVF or ICSI (each having their advocates, see chapter 11) is the usual preferred option in the fertility units that offer sperm antibody treatment, but intra-uterine insemination (IUI, see Figures 13 and 14, pages 200 and 202) is still an option that could be tried first. It is considerably cheaper and can be considered where clinically the sperm repeatedly fail to progress through the cervical mucus. It is, however, important that when attempting to 'wash away the antibodies' to ascertain that the sperm survive well (see page 206).

Prognosis

Specific therapies

Cervical mucus quality will certainly be improved by taking low-dose oestrogens, but results in terms of pregnancies achieved alone or with concomitant ovarian stimulation results have not been quantified. Even the efficacy of modern sperm antibody treatment is difficult to assess as washing is an integral part of semen preparation for all the ART treatments used. It is difficult to see if prognosis is altered at all by the antibodies being removed. However, where this is cited as the reason for the procedure, both IVF and ICSI seem to give similar pregnancy rates of around 30% – that is, no greater or less than for other indications for the use of ART (see chapter 11). The expected pregnancy rates in IUI overall, whatever the reason for its being utilised, are again around 15%.

The main value in considering the cervical region separately

Even for those who like myself believe the cervical region is worth investigating as a separate entity and consider that the PCT is one of the four key basic tests in the fertility profile, the presence of such a confused multi-factorial causative picture makes specific evaluation of data difficult. Similarly, instituting specific therapy when the PCT is repeatedly abnormal can be hard to justify.

A persistent negative PCT result rarely stays negative if the semen quality is reasonable and penetrative intercourse really is taking place. It has been demonstrated that many couples may have repeatedly negative tests (33%) but one in four of these still becomes pregnant. Only rarely do negative test results reflect a 'true cervical factor' presence (3%). Usually, the main reason for a negative first test is found to be iatrogenic (45%), with male or female factors – rather than the cervical factor – accounting for another 21%.

I believe that the main value in investigating the cervical region and including the PCT as a specific test in the fertility profile is that the underlying potential problem for the couple may present first here. In this regard psycho-sexual difficulties come specifically to mind.

The PCT can also help the couple by demonstrating the signs and time when intercourse is most likely to result in conception. While in a few cases, having intercourse to order may precipitate a coital problem, the chances of this are more than offset by the encouragement provided by a positive PCT result. This reinforces a couple's knowledge of themselves. There is a well-known positive placebo effect, with some 6% of couples in one study shown to have conceived following solely a PCT performed at the right time in the cycle.

All in all, coitus can be proven to be taking place and the value of investigating the cervical region specifically arguably very much outweighs the negatives as it adds complementary information to that from the other regions investigated. This helps complete a better understanding of the whole picture for the infertility team and couple.

Personal Comment

The trend nowadays in these 'cost effective' times is to equate the value of a test in infertility to pregnancy prediction. In this, the single PCT (post-coital test) falls down. Both positive and negative results correlate little with fertility outcome and can vary from month to month. If semen quality is reasonable, with normal coitus, eventually a positive result can usually be obtained. Also, psycho-sexual difficulties can be precipitated and the 'true cervical factor', if it exists at all, is rare. However, the PCT should not be consigned to history. It is still a useful monitor of sexual function and may indeed be the only way of detecting early a mechanical, coital or psycho-sexual problem. It examines the functioning of sperm that have been deposited inside the woman and her peri-ovular mucus quality, and is considered by some as one of the screening tests for an 'immunological' infertility factor. It has a positive placebo effect, promoting wellbeing in a couple and thus has the potential to initiate pregnancy. Provided its limitations are recognised and results compared with the rest of the fertility profile, and that back-up tests are done before any conclusions are drawn, it is still worth including PCTs for their valuable information-giving potential and their ability to identify for the believers the 'cervical factor' as a separate possible entity in the causation of infertility.

* * *

SECTION II: PHYSICAL COITAL PROBLEMS AND SEXUAL DYSFUNCTIONS

General points

Where there is a physical barrier or a psycho-sexual difficulty in one or both partners that prevents ejaculation in the vagina from taking place, infertility will almost invariably be the result. The problem may be primary (been there from the start) or secondary (developed later when previously all was well). Such problems may affect the male, the female or be shared. They are sometimes unique to the specific couple and not found with a change of partner. Dysfunction does not always lead to partner dissatisfaction and tension, but certainly can do.

Highlighting relevant physical anatomical defects does form part of this chapter but as a psycho-sexual dimension can arise even with a mechanically based difficulty, the focus is mainly on the psychological aspects. Indeed, whatever the reason, physical or psychological, and whether the problem has always been there or is new and/or temporary, psycho-sexual intervention may be helpful at some stage.

While not all couples with a mechanical barrier or a sexual dysfunction will be trying to conceive and may be satisfied in functioning sexually as they are, this next section, like the whole of the book itself, is written with those wanting conception in mind. It assumes a heterosexual relationship in which successful coitus is not happening but is desired and that, if enabled, would allow reproduction to progress on from that point. It also addresses what alternatives can then be considered if coitus is still not attained.

Alternative sexual preferences are not reviewed in this chapter as they fall outside the aim of this work, whose scope is confined to infertility (see chapter 11 for single sex pregnancy possibilities, page 197).

The basis of human sexuality

It is, I feel, helpful to have from the start an understanding of human sexuality, the mechanisms involved in coitus and the basic psychogenic approach to any related problems.

Sexual development is fundamental to our very existence. It is an ongoing process throughout our lives. There are normally six basic stages, starting during prenatal existence and developing onwards through to midlife and beyond. It is said that the adult phase, with the establishment of stable sexual relationship[s], is produced from the interweaving of the three separate developmental strands during childhood and adolescence. These are initially, sexual differentiation into male or female, sexual responsiveness and the capacity for close relationships.

Gender development can be manifested in seven different ways. These are chromosomal, gonadal, hormonal, internal sex organs, external sex organs, gender assigned at birth and personally assigned gender identity. Usually all match, giving a clear gender identity at birth of boy or girl. Embryonic gender development and assignment are more passive in the female than the male, where hormone production is required in the embryo to superimpose maleness upon the default position of femaleness.

Development in childhood depends initially on role-models, such as parents. Peer groups gradually become more influential and usually overt and covert sex education is part of a growing individual's environment. Gender identity in adolescence can be confusing, with pubertal changes in body shape, sex hormonal output and emotional instability. Sexuality becomes a very important aspect of gender.

Bio-rhythms in the female change more during development. There is a much greater degree of fluctuation in sex hormone output. As a consequence, greater swings can be seen in physical and psychological responses to this than in the male. This is most clearly seen during the menstrual cycle.

Sexual behaviour is ultimately controlled by the limbic system, sited in the brain stem, and other of the brain's higher centres. The majority of human sexuality functions are positive. It promotes reproduction of the species. Pair bonding, fostering intimacy and providing pleasure are important functions. Masculinity or femininity are asserted and act to reduce anxiety and tension. The negatives are the expression of hostility and material gain.

The primary male sexual response is clearly noticeable and focused but, in the female, it can remain hidden and involve not only the pelvic reproductive organs but also other parts of the body such as the breasts.

The male sexual response

The male sexual response has been divided into four phases by Masters and Johnson (1966). These are excitement leading to erection; secondly a plateau when lubrication and gland secretion takes place. Orgasm with emission and ejaculation then occurs. Lastly there is resolution, with detumescence (becomes soft again) and the resting (refractory) period.

The female sexual response

The lower vagina, clitoris and labia become engorged. Fluid appears in the vagina as a response to the increased blood supply and also from the pair of glands (Bartholin's glands) sited at the entrance to the vagina. All this is to facilitate penile entrance and make the area less hostile to sperm.

Unlike the male, where orgasm and ejaculation are the culmination and lead to a resting phase afterwards, in the human female, ejaculation is not usually noticeable, and orgasm is not inevitable. Indeed, the nature of female orgasm and its function remain the subject of much debate. It is not a pre-requisite for conception to occur in humans. The presence or absence of the 'G-spot' and whether it can be pinpointed by ultrasound as some claim is another red herring as far as conception is concerned.

Both men and women can remain sexual until death even at an advanced age as the basic events stay the same, with the ability to procreate staying to the end in the male. However, the bodily sexual response may differ at different times during the reproductive and mid-life phases and beyond. Sensuality can also alter, different senses predominating at different stages of life. It can become lessened by familiarity and heightened by change of circumstance.

Arousal and coital function control

In the male

In simple terms, penile erection (tumescence) depends on arterial blood filling a pair of cylindrical structures called the corpora cavernosa, which form most of the penis body. The flaccid resting state (detumescence) is achieved by the blood leaving the corpora cavernosa via veins and lymphatic drainage. Three sets of nerves are involved in the process. There is a local spinal reflex arc but, generally, control is through specific centres in the brain (mainly pre-optic hypothalamus oxytocin production), which can, in their turn, be over-ridden by higher brain centres.

Other genital tract organs, the prostate, seminal vesicles, bladder neck and urethra are involved in the generally linked processes of orgasm and ejaculation, together with local muscle responses (bulbo spongiosus). These are under reflex nerve control (see page 39).

The male sex hormone testosterone and its control mechanism play their part via the hypothalamic-pituitary axis. The names and functions are parallel to those previously described in the female (see chapter 9 and Figure 12, page 121).

In the female

There is also increased blood flow (vasocongestion) in the female sexual organs if she becomes sexually excited. It is less focused on a limited area and less visible as the reproductive organs are internal.

As in the male, control involves similar blood supply to deliver engorgement and sex hormones to stimulate the response. Nerve control may be by local reflexes but again these can be overridden by the brain and in turn its higher centres.

Male sexual dysfunction

It is not surprising that the incidence is unknown but it must run into many millions. Indeed, there can be few sexually active men who have not experienced a problem at some time or other, however transient it may have been. The culture one grows up in, religious values and teaching and the availability and usage or otherwise of sound advice/reassurance can also play a part. This is not only where the problem occurs in specific performance-demanding situations, but also where the problem has always been there or arrives later on but then becomes chronic. Erectile dysfunction is one of the commonest chronic medical disorders in men over 40 years of age. Male sexual interest (libido) and response, like the female, can decrease with age, illness or circumstance.

Main underlying causes in the male – mechanical and psychogenic

Anatomical
Anatomical abnormalities can include penile deformities, an over-tight foreskin and plaques developing on one side of the penis, causing a bend in it when aroused (Peyronie's disease). All these may lead to sexual dysfunction.

Vascular problems
Vascular problems (70%) are the commonest cause of male sexual dysfunction and are more likely to be found as age increases, especially in men with hypertension (33%), diabetes mellitus (70%), obesity and with high lipid (fasting cholesterol) levels. The blood flow to the penis, or venous outflow, is affected.

Essential drug treatment
Prescription drugs can be implicated. Anti-hypertensives may cause problems in up to 25% of men who take them, anti-psychotropic preparations in 50%. Beta-blockers and lithium (10%) are further such examples.

Nervous system disease
Brain tumours, infection and haemorrhage may all cause difficulty with arousal and coitus. So may nerve supply interference by diabetic neuropathy, and by diseases such as multiple sclerosis, Parkinsonism and dementia.

Mental illness
Mental illness includes diseases such as schizophrenia where 70% of men may have such problems. In overall fertility terms, although such illnesses can be rare, to the sufferer they are a significant cause.

Severing the nerve supply
Operations, especially in the rectal area, spinal cord lesions or spinal trauma can lead to erection and ejaculatory problems. Retrograde ejaculation may be the result – that is, the semen goes into the bladder instead of out via the penile urethra at ejaculation (see page 46).

Hormones
Congenital absence of the testicular cells that produce testosterone (Leydig cells), interference with male sex hormone production by drugs with an anti-androgen effect, and high levels of prolactin (hyperprolactinaemia) may cause sexual performance problems.

Lifestyle
Excessive alcohol and other similar risk factors such as smoking and non-prescribed drugs such as marijuana, cocaine, heroin and methadone can play their part in sexual dysfunction in both sexes but more especially the male. Fatigue, cramped living quarters, sharing with family that gives rise to embarrassment and lack of opportunities for spontaneous intimacy can also lead to such problems.

A psycho-sexual origin
Psycho-sexual problems account for the remainder of potential causes, sometimes in tandem with a mechanical factor, sometimes alone.

Diagnosis

History

Sexual problems may be spoken of for the first time in many different medical or counselling situations and not just when presenting with infertility. There may even have been an initial lack of awareness or a failure to admit that a problem exists until this is forced into the open by circumstances, such as can happen when infertility is being investigated – for example, when semen analysis (chapter 7) or a post-coital test (see page 137) is called for. However, when the problem is discovered, whatever discipline is involved and whatever the classification given, taking a comprehensive history of the problem is paramount. By itself, this can guide the health professional as to the likelihood of the cause being mechanical or there being a psycho-sexual dimension as well or instead. For example, 30-50% of diabetics have erectile problems and, as with other illnesses, there may also be resultant low sexual desire. Overwork and the fatigue of modern lifestyles where couples seldom meet is a physical cause but may also give rise to loss of desire. Self-esteem and confidence are often low. Symptoms of depression may become evident.

Physical examination and tests

Physical examination and tests, coupled with the history, may determine alone whether a general or specific physical/mechanical situation is present that may be amenable to appropriate surgical or medical therapy, or that there is a psycho-sexual problem. For example, physical examination of the genital area may reveal deformities or the absence of vital organs. Vascular, infective, hormonal or nervous disease require confirmatory examinations and tests specific to what is suspected.

Male treatment and prognosis

No direct therapy available

Sometimes nothing can be offered where a physical reason for the sexual dysfunction and infertility is present. It cannot always be reversed as the damage may be too great or untreatable. This can particularly be the case with some vascular and nerve diseases or physical damage situations. It may also be unwise in general health terms to alter a drug therapy regime even where it is a causative factor.

Lifestyle changes

Lifestyle changes are important, although one partner giving up the job that could be a factor may not be warranted. Smoking, drinking excessive amounts of caffeine and alcohol and lifestyle drugs should be stopped. Cholesterol levels may need to be normalised.

Surgery and mechanical

These approaches to achieving erections and coitus include vacuum devices to fit on the penis, penile silicone implants, the removal of Peyronie's disease plaques plus vascular surgery for venous leaks and arterial flow problems, but none of these is ideal. Vacuums have a transient effect, the tumescence created being kept in place by a penile ring. Bruising may also occur because of trauma when placing such items in situ in what may then become a very engorged vascular area. An implant creates a semi-erection allowing coitus. Straightening the penis, as in men with Peyronie's disease, shortens it.

Circumcision may be the answer to painful erections and coitus if the foreskin is very tight or when it does not retract easily or at all.

Medical therapies

The most dramatic advance has been oral drug therapy, which is now much used, although mostly for recreational purposes and not in the infertility situation. There are two groups of drugs. Neither causes an erection but either can improve the quality of one. One group (apomorphines) work centrally as a dopamine-agonist in the pituitary gland (Uprima) (see chapter 9, page 126). The other group act locally at genital level. This group includes yohimbine (20% effective), which has been marketed for years (see chapter 12) and sildenafil citrate (phosphodiesterase-5-inhibitors). This latter was the first of this recent fortuitously developed and highly researched family of preparations (70% find it effective). But, in studies, placebo has been found to have an effect in 50% as well. It should be noted that a number of alternatives within this family are now available in addition to sildenafil.

There have also been significant advances in both 'trans-urethral' and 'intracorporeal' self-administered drugs containing prostaglandin E1. 'Trans-urethral' signifies the preparation is inserted into the urine exit hole of the penis; this has been been noted to work within seven minutes in 65% of men. 'Intracorporeal' signifies the vasoactive (improves vascularisation) drug is self-injected into the body of the penis; this is successful in producing an erection that lasts for up to 45 minutes in 65% of men.

Spinal injury treatment at present involves the use of vibrators, electro-ejaculation, or testicular biopsy techniques to try to obtain semen for AI or IVF/ICSI. However, prognosis is often poor as quality semen production requires reasonably frequent ejaculation to sustain it. (See also chapter 7, Retrograde ejaculation, page 46).

Hormone treatments

As in the female, where ovulation can be stimulated (see page 126), dopamine agonists are highly effective in the male for treating 'hyperprolactinaemia'. This hormone can influence gonadal function but unlike in the female where ovulation can be disturbed with hyperprolactinaemia, in the male it is more usually associated with erectile difficulties. The presence of a possible causative brain tumour needs to be eliminated first.

Hypogonadism may cause testosterone deficiency and lead to loss of libido and to impotence. Testosterone patches can be effective in the former but in the latter may switch off relevant pituitary function, erection control and sperm production by an excess feed-back effect.

Iatrogenic

Where the cause is brought about by investigations or treatment such as a PCT (see page 137), unless the information to be provided by a test is essential, to persist is wrong. It runs the risk of the problem spilling over into relationships at home. However, if it is essential to obtain a semen sample pre-IVF, the stress of having to do so can be reduced by making freezing/advanced storage available so that there can some flexibility over timing (see chapter 11, page 214).

The psychotherapeutic approach to management

General information

Six different groupings of psycho-sexual dysfunction are recognised in the male. The incidence of these can differ markedly even between close neighbours such as the UK and Ireland. These are:
- inhibited sexual desire/loss of libido (UK 4%, Ireland 34%)
- premature ejaculation (UK 34%, Ireland 11%)
- delayed (retarded) ejaculation (UK 9%, Ireland3%)
- ejaculatory pain (very rare)
- sexual phobias (very rare)
- erectile dysfunctions/impotence (UK 48%, Ireland 10%)

Erectile dysfunction, the last on the list, is the commonest presenting problem that causes infertility, although all the above can be implicated.

There is often an unclear divide between psychological and physical factors. Psychotherapy may be appropriate for both men and women as an additive to treating a physical cause that has been detected by history and examination. It is the therapy of choice where a psychogenic origin is the most likely single cause. Wherever the initial disclosure is made, the interest of the relevant health professionals and the facilities available will determine whether the problem can be dealt with locally or will need to be referred to a specialised psychotherapy clinic.

In this latter situation, a multidisciplinary, mutually respectful service is the ideal treatment environment. This involves trained sexual counsellors working with gynaecologists, urologists and psychiatrists interested in the area. A tertiary care infertility clinic may well have such expertise in house.

In infertility, referral for specialised psychotherapy counselling should be easy and fast and appointments made via any involved health worker. It is not only doctors who are the first point of disclosure of such problems. You should expect facilities and staff to be welcoming, discreet and as stress free as possible. Sometimes spontaneous cures occur (explained by the placebo effect), and attention to an underlying disease process may result in resolution.

Psychotherapy for specific sexual dysfunctions is specialised in its own right and worth discussing in further detail. It consists of an initial interview to define the problem and set goals. The therapy then becomes two-pronged. A psychodynamic approach is taken by the counsellor to any problems or causes that are revealed. As the story unfolds and providing the sexual dysfunction has been identified clearly, behavioural therapy also commences. This is modified according to which category the sexual dysfunction falls into and to whether it is primary, secondary or situational.

The basics are described for both men and women. The former is considered here first. In the context of infertility, any differences in women are dealt with in the section on female sexual dysfunction that follows this.

The initial interview, assessment and goal setting

Psycho-sexual intervention will always start with a personalised diagnostic interview and assessment by the therapist. This is usually a fully trained, qualified, experienced sex and relationships counsellor or Psychiatrist. Tertiary care units should either have the former on the staff or be known to them for referral.

The couple are assessed as to their basic knowledge of the relevant anatomy and physiology, but focusing on the current problem. Is it primary or secondary, situational or conditional (particular circumstances) and what is the duration? Desire, expectations and potential myths about sexual functioning are explored and whether there is a partnership disorder as well. In such a case, relationship counselling is also necessary before the sexual problem can be addressed; otherwise any sex therapy instituted will inevitably be sabotaged.

The goals of therapy are determined by the therapist and client(s) together at or after the initial diagnostic interview.

Psychodynamic counselling

A psychodynamic approach is taken to treatment. The idea is to create through discussion some level of understanding as to what is causing the trouble. This often may take a number of sessions. In the case of infertility, some may need to be held solo and the rest jointly with the partner. There may be fears or problems with the tests being demanded of a couple in the infertility setting – requiring a man to produce a semen sample in inappropriate pressurised surroundings is particularly likely to cause trouble as is the pressure of having to have coitus to someone else's order, for example for a PCT. On the other hand, 'permission giving' for sexual relations to start may be needed, say after an illness or for a new relationship starting after the death of a previous partner. Problems of desire are often mixed up with erectile dysfunction. This may be revealed as the real cause. Hidden causes may be discovered, such as chemical dependence, psychiatric illness, couple disharmony or disagreement about wanting children. It maybe necessary to work through resistance or blocks that have built up over the years.

Behavioural therapy

Behavioural therapy is usually based on the educational and psychotherapeutic modules originally developed by Masters and Johnson in the 1960s. It aims to develop a relationship initially from a sensual to a sexual one. In all male infertility cases, the partner is involved in the exercises. Throughout, as the couple progress with their 'homework', feedback is given to the therapist as part of a two-way exchange of information. Joint 'sensate focus exercises' start with non-sexual touch, progressing to sexual arousal, erection, coitus and controlled ejaculation.

Specific techniques are used to deal with particular problems posed by the different dysfunctions. These include teaching the partner stop/start or squeeze techniques for premature ejaculation. Penile stimulation techniques can be employed for ejaculatory failure where the aim is to obtain semen for insemination (see chapter 11, page 203). Vibrators may also be a help if this is the aim.

Low desire is more difficult to treat than erectile dysfunction but the approach to both is similar. A combination of a self-focus programme for the man and an initial ban on coitus for the couple is often used. Relaxation and fantasy exercises are encouraged to enable the man to be comfortable with his own body and subsequently with his partner.

It is best if these programmes are carried out without the added stress of trying to conceive for a few months. However, there may be situations where the desire for pregnancy is such that couples want to continue to try to conceive. Age and duration of infertility may play a part in this.

The concomitant use of drugs (such as sildenafil, or similar) that influence erectile quality, as detailed above, may sometimes help to break a vicious circle and can be considered.

Prognosis in male sex therapy

Where a psycho-sexual approach is the primary method of treatment, in terms of infertility itself, success rates are confused and difficult to interpret. Infertility has many confounding variables but if there is nothing physically wrong, and therapy gets coitus started, there should be a normal chance of conception.

When the goal of therapy is achieving coitus, the outcome is more favourable in some psycho-sexual groupings than others. Overall, around 30% have a successful outcome. Erectile dysfunction seems to be associated with the best chance of success. Sixty-five per cent of men can be expected to succeed in having coitus if the programme is completed. Success in overcoming premature ejaculation runs at around 40% in most programmes.

If couples still wish to give every chance to achieving a conception during 'sensate focusing' treatment, samples of sperm can be collected and DIY artificial insemination (AI) can be utilised (see chapter 11, pages 203 and 205), although this can interfere with steps in the psychotherapeutic regime. Results better than those normally associated with AI can be expected if all else is otherwise normal.

When the treatment fails, and couples do not manage to start successful coitus, again if reasonable quality samples can be produced, AI or IUI can be discussed together with IVF. The last resorts are AID (donor insemination) or surgical testicular/epididymal sperm recovery followed by IVF or ICSI (see chapter 11, page 212).

Main causes of mechanical dysfunction in women

Congenital blockages

The inability to have intercourse may be mechanical due to absence or a congenital blockage in the vagina, occasionally by an over-tight or imperforate hymen but more often by the vagina being divided into two parts by a septum (Figure 6, page 66). Effective coitus may be impossible while these circumstances remain.

Acquired genital tract blockages

Scarring leading to vaginal deformities may occur following operations or infection in the area. Alternatively, vulvo/vaginal cysts may cause a problem; these can give rise to pain on intercourse ('dyspareunia') and this can lead to the cessation of coital activity.

Pain may be sited at the entrance to the vagina (superficial dyspareunia); this is usually associated with lack of arousal, scarring infection or cysts. Deep dyspareunia is felt at the top of the vagina on deep penetration or penile thrusting and is usually due to internal pelvic disease such as endometriosis, tumours or infection (PID, see chapter 8, pages 78-9).

Dyspareunia should be differentiated from vaginismus, which is not a physical disability or disease but an emotional condition with psychogenic causes that manifest themselves in a physical response.

Psycho-sexual problems in women

In women, five sexual dysfunctions are recognised: inhibited sexual desire; orgasmic dysfunction; dyspareunia (superficial and deep); sexual phobias; and vaginismus. However, infertility will only result where coitus is prevented or stops, as in vaginismus or sometimes with dyspareunia.

Inhibited sexual desire (what used to be called frigidity), resulting either from lack of sexual interest or impaired arousal, is the commonest category, accounting for some 50% of cases overall, though not in the infertility situation. This inhibition may be situational and early life experiences may play a part; equally, it may be due to failure of physiological responses during sexual arousal. Using 'lifestyle' drugs may sometimes also be involved as may female genital mutilation practices banned by the World Health Organisation and many countries.

Orgasmic dysfunction is also a common complaint today (20% of clients), but is not found as much in the infertile (only 10%). The problem may be total or situational, primary or secondary and, unless intercourse stops as a result, does not cause infertility.

Sexual phobias. A small number of women will complain of sexual phobias such as an aversion to genital touching or seminal fluid themselves. This in itself may, however, not cause infertility unless coitus stops.

Dyspareunia is the fourth dysfunction listed and is the term used to describe painful or difficult intercourse. It may be experienced at the vaginal entrance (superficial) or deep inside (deep) and has an organic cause. It needs to be differentiated from...

Vaginismus, the final complaint, which can occur in up to 20% of the general female population at some time. It is the most common sexual dysfunction found in the infertility setting (34%). Sexual intercourse is either impossible or so painful that the muscles surrounding the entrance to the vagina automatically contract when penetration is attempted. The woman feels she has no control over this but other sexual responses may be normal. It can be mild or severe and, in the infertile, situational, related to or precipitated by anxiety over the situation and the treatments being used. The majority of vaginismus in infertility is primary (no successful intercourse ever).

Treatment and prognosis in women

Physical blockage

Congenital and/or acquired blockage should be suspected in women with a history of amenorrhoea (no periods) or dyspareunia. In some cases, after a confirmatory physical examination, reconstructive surgery can be offered. Where indicated, results can be excellent but psycho-sexual counselling may be needed as well. Such surgery should be used only where appropriate and not with vaginismus. In the past operations to widen the vaginal entrance were used for this but these may well worsen the problem and fail to address the underlying psychogenic issue.

Psycho-sexual difficulties

General

In this case the presenting cause of the infertility is usually vaginismus and the approach is psychotherapeutic. The basics of investigation and treatment for this remain the same as in the male. The same personnel, facilities and approach are involved, modified to suit the female. At the initial history-taking session, goals are established jointly with the therapist and a verbal contract agreed. Treatment involves an exploration of the problem as seen by the couple with the therapist. A psychodynamic approach and accompanying behavioural therapy are again used. The length of treatment will vary depending on the severity of the problem and whether it is situational, or primary or secondary. Sessions are usually together, although one or two may need to be solo if requested.

The aim of therapy is not just being able to tolerate full penetrative intercourse without severe pain and anxiety and thus potentially cure a cause for infertility; it is also about understanding what lies behind the body's resistance, why it is saying 'no' and what 'yes' entails. The structured approach that is recommended has three main purposes:

- to (re)build a sexual relationship;
- to gain insight by identifying causes;
- to learn specific techniques that will make a recurrence less likely and easier to cope with.

Behavioural therapy for women

To attain the goals listed above, again as with men, the therapist first takes the woman's history and then follows a two-pronged psycho-dynamic approach together with more formal behavioural therapy. Again this is over a number of very regular (every 1-2 weeks) arranged sessions for both partners. A detailed follow-up of the history of both continues to be taken during these sessions, each separately.

Behavioural therapy treatment for vaginismus often starts with a self-sensate focus programme for the woman, in which she concentrates alone on her own body and how she feels about it. When she is comfortable about this, the couple start initially with non-genital touching exercises. This 'homework' builds gradually (the time needed depends on how favourable the response is) to becoming genitally focused. The exercises differ anatomically but not in principle from those for men, going on to gradual vaginal containment (finger put and kept inside) by self and then using the partner's fingers, progressing on to tampons and subsequently vaginal trainers, upwards from the smallest eventually to penis entry. Relaxation methods are also taught; fantasy may also be included.

When success is achieved, contraception is often advised until at least the six-week follow-up date. This is because if pregnancy occurs too soon and coitus stops again, as it does with some couples, the necessary reinforcement of regular coitus may not occur.

The other causes of female sexual dysfunction may be principally treated in a similar manner to this psychogenic approach to vaginismus as well as attending to underlying physical precipitating factors.

Prognosis of sex therapies in women

During treatment, women usually cope well with the pressures and couples stay 'together' in their relationship unless the cracks are already there. Where treatment is completed, full success can be expected in some 85% of women. In overall terms, with a sexual problem on her side only, the majority of infertile women (82%) complete the prescribed course and achieve coitus. Over 30% may achieve pregnancy soon after.

Joint sexual problems

Incidence

It is now well recognised that in over one third of couples presenting to a sex and relationship service, a male sex dysfunction turns out to be accompanied by a female one or vice versa. Any combination may occur, sometimes the same, sometimes different. For example, a loss of desire can be common to both, and ejaculatory problems may lead to loss of desire or orgasm.

Often the fact that both have such difficulties is evident from the start, but one problem may mask the presence of the other. A therapist may discover, for instance, that in trying to achieve success in a man with erectile difficulties, vaginismus may be revealed in the partner, or the converse may happen when vaginismus treatment is a success.

Cause

Why this happens is unclear. Either the problem was always there, or it is now being precipitated by performance anxiety. It may be associated with natural selection in a partnership of like for like. There can be lack of communication between the two on sexual matters, ignorance or indifference to the need to be sexual as part of being human. History taking may reveal one partner as being the type who is fearful or unwilling to push the other on sexual matters if there has been an initial problem or rebuff.

Treatment and prognosis

If a problem is revealed early on in the other partner as well, a 'behavioural therapy' type approach is usually beneficial, modified in each case to the dysfunction type. This will sometimes involve simultaneous treatment for both and on other occasions the partners will be separated from each other. However, if the revelation occurs after successfully treating one partner, the difficulty is to sustain what has been achieved while working on the other appropriately. Excellent inter-partner communication and encouragement are essential for success.

Personal Comment

> *To be sexual, intimate and satisfied does not necessarily*
> *require penetrative sex. On the other hand, conception can*
> *occur whether or not normal sexuality is present, providing*
> *coitus is not inhibited by an obstruction. Without some form*

of real shared intimacy, however, a couple's relationship can become problematic and unsatisfying. Considerable shame and anxiety are still associated with sexual dysfunction and many couples find it difficult to admit they have a potential psychological problem. The motivation of wanting a child may force acknowledgment after sometimes many years of non-consummation and distress. To wait so long is a pity as results of therapy in expert hands are excellent.

SECTION III: STRESS

Background

Stress may be defined as an excessive demand upon physical or mental energy. It is normal for humans to feel stressed upon occasion, sometimes even overly so. But, when the specific situational stress response starts to affect, and possibly interfere with, normal life functioning, this is excessive and needs to be dealt with.

Not all of us become stressed by the same things and reactions may be visible or hidden, differing from person to person. Some appear better able to cope than others, possibly because of a less negative perception of stressful stimuli. It is widely accepted now that at least 25% of infertile couples have recognisable manifestations of stress. These are more likely to be visible in the woman and hidden in the man.

There is a close relationship between the physiological and the psychological. Control of the stress response is via psycho-neuro-endocrine pathways, including the main hormonal interactions that control gonadal function. Substances such as adrenalin (now known as epinephrine), noradrenalin, serotonin and melatonin are produced that act directly in the brain. Gonadotrophin and prolactin hormones are released from the pituitary gland; these influence the menstrual cycle and ovulation (see chapter 9, page 108 and Figure 12, page 121).

It is said that behavioural responses and hormone release patterns seem to differ, depending on whether the reaction is to a threat stress (solely protective) or to a stress associated with sexual activity (preservation of the species). The neuro-endocrine response in the latter is more widespread across the whole area of emotion control.

Why infertility? Reasons for excessive stress

From the earliest of times, infertility has been documented as a stressful situation. However, life is itself highly stressful and the part stress plays in the genesis of infertility is unclear. It has not been proven how stress generally or specifically contributes to failure to conceive or lowers the prognosis of therapy. Excessive stress has, however, been linked to menstrual and ovulation problems. It can cause coital difficulties, and tubal spasm has been reported. But in only 5% of couples is an emotional abnormality thought to be truly linked to infertility.

To be fruitful and multiply, with infertility accepted as grounds for divorce, is still the norm in many societies. The vast majority of couples wish to have a family at some time or other. When it does not happen as planned, this is perceived as a problem to which feeling stressed is a natural reaction. Often such couples are high achievers in other areas and failure, possibly for the first time in their lives, can be hard to cope with. The couple realise that this failure can result in loss of control over that most highly personal area – their sex life. To this can be added the stress-provoking atmosphere of expectancy from family and friends.

The process of diagnosis and treatment may make it worse. An excessively formal clinic organised according to a narrow medical model with a rigid ambience, absence of necessary facilities and privacy, and failure to keep the couple in the picture as members of the team that are helping them may contribute to a stressful atmosphere whose presence may not be acknowledged. Indeed, sometimes the clinical staff themselves feel stressed in what is not always a tranquil work setting and this can be passed on to the couple.

While intentional childlessness is on the increase and acceptable in our society, worldwide it is not yet accepted that infertility can be considered as a form of 'natural selection' or to object to its being treated on the basis that the world is overpopulated. Infertility is, however, sadly a Cinderella subject when public health provision is discussed, even though it can affect and distress up to one in six to eight couples.

Emotional responses to infertility

It is necessary to take into account family values, cultural norms and comfort with one's own sexuality as these will influence an individual's pattern of reaction and coping mechanisms. Most infertile couples follow a well-recognised pattern. There is initially surprise followed by denial, anger, isolation, guilt, and finally acceptance or resolution.

In the past, this pathway was felt by psychologists to be linked to 'neuroticism', with the neurotic personality-type being more predisposed to respond quicker and more intensely, especially if female. However, it is now accepted that the male may be deliberately concealing his depth of feeling and be just as stressed as his partner.

Infertility can be perceived by individuals or couples as involving significant personal loss. It touches on relationships, health, status or prestige, self-esteem, self-confidence, security, fantasy or hope of fulfilling an important fantasy, as well as the loss of something of great symbolic value. It is hardly surprising that a reactive depression-like state can envelope those failing to conceive. This is more likely to happen if they become isolated and hide away, avoiding others with children, or when progress towards resolution is slow or arrested. A grieving process, which can be very painful, will aid resolution. This does not mean that the wish to be fertile and trying for a child has to cease, but working through it can free the couple from the psychological millstone of childlessness.

Diagnosis

History

Often no specific history is volunteered by those who appear to the clinic staff to be responding particularly emotionally. As discussed earlier in this chapter, psycho-sexual problems may become manifest. Disorganisation, distraction, envy, fatigue, obsessions, headaches and irritability are symptoms and signs that can be noted with increased frequency in those attending infertility services. In many clinics these signs have to be relied upon as the sole acknowledgment that a couple are suffering excessive stress that may need attention.

Such manifestations of stress need to be differentiated from serious psycho-pathological problems that may need expert psychiatric trained personnel to diagnose and treat.

Physical examination

Physical examination is likely to be inconclusive. Increased heart rate and blood pressure are expected findings but these are not specific to infertility consultations or couples.

Investigations

Hormonal and psychological diagnostic tools are available, but it is true to say they are sadly only likely to be encountered by patients in clinics with a special interest in stress and its effects.

Hormone tests

The secretory patterns of hormones alter with stress, but not all are detectable. Women exhibit greater fluctuations than men, with alterations in adrenalin (now called epinephrine), nor-adrenalin and cortisol all being shown to correlate with excessively stressed infertile individuals. Prolactin is usually routinely tested in the female as part of investigating her menstrual cycle. Mild intermittent elevations (stress spikes, see chapter 9) have been linked to stress and ovulatory difficulty. A minimum of four blood samples taken at different times is considered necessary to sustain such a diagnosis (see page 119).

The menstrual cycle itself is, however, seldom affected by stress spikes. The contribution to infertility may instead be via an effect on the luteal phase of the cycle and on progesterone, interfering with the positive feedback of pulsatile GnRH or vital receptors (see pages 108-9).

Psychological tests

Psychological tests have been used by behavioural scientists to measure emotion for many years. Many self-report questionnaires have been created and utilised in the infertility setting. Scoring systems have been devised to try to differentiate findings from similarly tested fertile couples (controls) so as to see who really needs treatment and to monitor its effects. New tests are invented regularly.

The better questionnaires are flexible enough to allow language to be modified to suit the local situation and include ways of testing 'faking good'. This has been used to 'out' the male as being just as stressed-out an individual as his partner.

The majority, but not all, studies have shown infertile patients to be more stressed than fertile controls. Indeed, when stress levels have been measured against such controls, both hormonally and psychologically, there has not been universal agreement that infertile couples are more stressed than anyone else in society confronted by the problems of everyday life.

Therapy

Prevention

Social attitudes and practices need to change if the stress laid by society upon the infertile couple is to be lessened.

At the clinic level, stress-provoking situations need to be minimised. A planned approach is needed with as little repetition as possible. The couple must themselves be made to feel an intimate part of the management team. Education as to what is going on from the start helps achieve this and to de-stress. Adherence to appointment times by both sides helps.

Some measure of control is necessary and supervision is important, but the pace of investigations and treatment wherever possible should be chosen by the couple. Periods of reflection before embarking on a change in therapy are useful and maximise possible expected placebo effects.

Setting a limit of time or number of goes for a specific treatment is wise. Nothing is more soul-destroying and stressful than continuing the same unsuccessful therapy year after year. However, setting a time limit on attendance itself can be stress-making and counterproductive. Encouraging second opinions can also be important.

A policy of helping to counsel-out (stop any further active investigations or treatment) at a certain moment, as judged by the clinic, should always be there. For couples who voluntarily discontinue, they should be made aware that an open-door policy operates should they wish to return later.

Overall, in terms of the clinic's general operation, stress can be minimised and anxiety lowered to great effect. The multidisciplinary staff must demonstrate by their actions that they appreciate how stressful infertility and the associated procedures are for most people.

Personal initiatives

The couple themselves may attempt to keep the stress under control by employing counter-distractions or seek to share experiences with others by joining for a time an independent self-help infertility support group or internet chat line (see pages 257-8).

Psychologically-based stress management

The counsel of perfection for psychological stress management is for couples to be given access to suitably trained infertility counsellors. Using specific techniques the couple can be helped to cope with the symptoms of guilt, anger, frustration and isolation and also later on be given help to embark on the grieving process necessary to achieving resolution. The practical support, education and counselling provided gives opportunities for patients to develop positive perceptions.

Psychotherapeutic interventions

Psychotherapeutic interventions may be helpful to deal with specific emotional difficulties, either as a solo couple or in a group setting. Relaxation therapies are available in a number of forms (see below and also chapter 12, page 248) including yoga, transcendental meditation or autogenic training. Some may find these of positive benefit generally or to help cope with a specific treatment that proves to be more distressing than others. IVF is considered one of these particularly stressful experiences as it is perceived by most infertile couples to be the end of the line.

Pharmacotherapy

Few doctors would quarrel with a patient using some form of relaxation therapy. However, they themselves are invariably trained to treat with drugs and 'patients' seem usually to like to have a remedy prescribed for them. While the stress response can be modified by drugs with tranquillising or sedative actions, these are not the answer in infertility except very temporarily in an emergency pathological-stress situation. They may alter hormonal production, hinder conception, affect an early pregnancy and lead to dependency.

A mix of two ovulation induction agents (see chapter 9, page 124), clomiphene citrate and bromocriptine, has been found effective where mild stress spikes of prolactin are present in the absence of any other cause for the infertility ('unexplained infertility').

Prognosis

Prophylaxis

Many of the general steps taken in a clinic's attempts to lessen stress in infertility are commonsense and just good practice. They can sometimes be difficult to implement in a very busy out-patient setting dealing with all problems and not just infertility. Their effect has not been formally measured but certainly it is the experience of many in the field that compliance with management usually seems better. Some indication as to their possible benefit on stress can, however, be gleaned from data seen in the IVF setting where pre-treatment attendence with a fertility counsellor was compulsory. For instance, the quality of semen, thought to be a casualty of excessive stress in IVF, did not, in the author's clinic where pre-treatment counselling was compulsory for all IVF attendees, appear to be impaired on the day of oocyte recovery compared with the initial sample.

In the same clinic the number of couples with decreased psychological coping scores as compared with controls, seemed to lessen when measured after the IVF therapy. The achievement of pregnancy or otherwise has not, however, been linked to this. This perhaps suggests that recommended measures to manage general stress do pay off in terms of patient wellbeing, and to have formal counselling as part of all IVF programmes therefore seems worthwhile, but does not improve pregnancy rates, at least in IVF.

Psychologically based stress management

Relaxation therapies, of which transcendental meditation and autogenic training are two of the most used, have been shown now by a number of authorities, including the author, to be associated with a fall in both hormonal and psychological marker levels in women but a rise in men, though men's hormones normally fluctuate much less. This finding has been interpreted as showing that the man initially fakes the psychological responses but as he relaxes he starts to tell the truth.

It is more difficult to measure the influence of such therapy on pregnancy rates, although a spontaneous conception rate of 42% was found after autogenic training in couples with a mean length of infertility of 5.5 years. This study was, however, uncontrolled.

Pharmacotherapy

Where stress spikes of prolactin are found in the woman in a couple who are otherwise apparently normal, I found a mixture of clomiphene citrate and bromocriptine to be significantly better than placebo (31% versus only 2.5%) in promoting pregnancy.

Personal Comment

Fertility should not be equated with success and infertility with failure. Survival of the species is a basic instinct but procreation need not be considered as the only measure of relationship fulfilment. Life itself is stressful and it is not surprising that many infertile couples feel stress in their situation. Not all admit they are bothered about having difficulty in conceiving, but in reality they have to be or they would not be putting themselves through sometimes difficult investigations and treatment. Positive benefits accrue when staff recognise stress is an underlying factor in infertility, try to minimise their part in its genesis and discourage isolationism from pressurising families and friends. Stress is a normal reaction but you need to be freed when it becomes abnormal and incessant.

SECTION IV: UNEXPLAINED INFERTILITY

What is 'unexplained infertility'?

Medicine is full of words that are used to conceal diagnostic inadequacies such as 'idiopathic', 'essential' and 'unexplained'. These tags suggest a specific underlying cause is present but in reality they hide the fact that none has actually been discovered.

'Unexplained infertility' is therefore not a diagnosis of cause for infertility at all. It simply means that either nothing really is wrong, or that when the present available tests are carried out they are not good enough to find out what the problem is.

This leads to distress in patients who, if not pre-counselled that this can happen, cannot understand why, and an inexperienced health professional may equally feel uneasy and inadequate in these circumstances. In the future, greater understanding and better tests may help diminish the number of couples labelled as 'unexplained infertile', but, at present, at least 20% of couples are likely be told after investigations have been completed that they have 'unexplained infertility'.

'Cause'

Consideration of only some of the potential inadequacies in the basic fertility profile (see chapter 6, page 32), in semen analysis, the post-coital test, hormonal function tests and laparoscopy, soon shows why the label 'unexplained infertility' is applied to so many couples.

So little of male function is capable of being tested beyond routine semen analysis and basic hormonal control. For instance, what is a normal sperm? How is it that ICSI can still work with non-mature and apparently morphologically abnormal sperm? Why does conception still occur in so many with negative PCTs? And what is the role of sperm antibodies?

It is possible to test for ovulation in the overall sense and whether it is happening. However, exact detection of ovulation and abnormalities in the phases of the menstrual cycle are difficult to diagnose with certainty and results can vary from month to month (see also the NaProTechnology section below). It is also unclear why, even when ovulation and coitus appear to coincide with no other abnormality, conception may still not occur.

In the uterus, the secrets behind implantation and its failure are slowly but surely being unravelled but it cannot yet be routinely tested. We do not know why some women have no difficulty conceiving in the presence of significant amounts of fibroids and endometriosis while others do. The patency (openness) of the fallopian tubes can be tested satisfactorily in a number of ways but other associated bio-physical functions of the tubes, such as hormonal and other local secretions, cannot.

To all this uncertainty can be added the potential effects of stress and the interaction of differing fertility potentials coming together. Some partners appear to be able to compensate for minor inadequacies in the other, some not.

Last but not least, we do not understand how and when the placebo effect will work.

How to minimise the incidence of 'unexplained infertility'

The number of couples labelled as having unexplained infertility is certainly dependent on a number of factors that good practice can address:

- good quality control in the laboratory responsible for hormonal and semen analysis tests;
- appropriate facilities, skills, expertise, training and experience in assessing the tubal factor by ultrasound, X-ray imaging and/or surgery;
- using laparoscopy instead of X-ray or ultrasound to assess tubal factors. This has been shown by the WHO to cut the incidence of unexplained infertility from nearly 50% to 20%. Without it, endometriosis and peri-tubal adhesions can be missed;

- always repeating at least one or more times any abnormal laboratory test before a diagnosis is confirmed.

It has also been shown that repeating the fertility profile fully can halve
the incidence of unexplained infertility, bringing it down to a hard core
of some 10% of couples. This is impractical for most and can be very
stressful and frustrating except where couples have expressly sought a
second opinion.

Treatment and prognosis

Doing nothing

In couples with unexplained infertility, the situation is often one of a lower fertility potential than normal rather than total inability. The average
cycle fecundity (potential reproductive capacity per cycle) of such couples who eventually conceive has been found to be higher in those who
conceive spontaneously than in those for whom some intervention was
prescribed empirically (3.8% versus 1.8%). Given time, many couples
labelled as having unexplained infertility will eventually conceive (the
placebo effect), sometimes even after the couple have long given up.

An individual's chance of eventually conceiving without therapy
with a specific partner cannot be estimated with much accuracy and it
alters with age. In the female, it is accepted that the cumulative pregnancy rate falls some 2% per year over 25 years of age and 2% per
month after she is over 40.

To do nothing for, say, some six months provided investigations have
been completed in a timely fashion is optimal advice when nothing has
been found. Six months is not written in stone and could be more if the
woman is under 35 years of age and less if over. A firm date for review
should be given when this period starts. It is worth noting that in one
study which followed up couples with unexplained infertility over eight
years, I found 46% had at least one pregnancy, 61% of which occurred
in a cycle without active therapy of any kind.

While most couples are willing to accept the advice of an agreed short-term pause without treatment, other options may need to be considered. The statistical argument that within eight years pregnancy will eventually arrive in almost 50% of such couples is hardly acceptable to a couple who may have already waited a long time.

Self-help

Non-medical approaches, including prayer, visits to shrines, diets, counselling and relaxation, have all been known anecdotally to succeed, as have vaginal and scrotal douches. They usually do no harm and may help relieve stress.

Pregnancies have been known occasionally to occur spontaneously after adoption. This has been examined but not found to be of positive therapeutic value.

Medically based treatments

The desire for pregnancy can be so compelling that many couples request some form of therapy no matter how ill-founded, illogical or empirical (not based upon scientific reasoning) many past studies have shown it may be. Great pressure can be brought to bear on the clinician to support this. When active treatment is used it is possible that it only brings forward something that was going to happen in any case.

Many alternatives have been suggested including muscle relaxants, antibiotics and alternative therapies such as herbal medicines and acupuncture (see chapter 12, pages 249-50). The majority, however, try to concentrate on ensuring ovulation takes place and, if possible, that its timing coincides with coitus. But, at best, as stated below, in the few situations where proper studies have taken place, results are similar to those for a placebo.

Ovarian stimulation

As noted in chapter 9 in the section on ovulation induction (page 128), ovarian stimulation is widely used – and abused in situations such as 'unexplained infertility'. In particular, anti-oestrogens such as clomiphene citrate are prescribed, administered monthly, or in alternate months as their effect seems to last for such a period of time. The rationale is solely one of 'to be sure to be sure' ovulation occurs. Placebo-controlled study data showing that the use of ovarian stimulation in unexplained infertility is unjustified, are seemingly ignored. With or without an injection of hCG to simulate the LH surge to time ovulation (chapter 9, page 124), the number of pregnancies achieved is no better than with placebo, yet there is a significant side-effect potential.

Bromocriptine has also been used in this way but, except in the presence of stress spikes and in combination with clomiphene citrate, despite a positive trend, it did not perform statistically significantly better than placebo (29% versus 8.6%).

Artificial insemination (AIH/Partner)

Artificial insemination (AI) using the partner's (husband's: AIH) semen alone, deposited intra-vaginally or cervically, has also been used again just to try *something*. In one study some years ago in a London hospital by the author, of some 400 cervico/vaginal AIs in 34 patients, four conceived, but three of these in a cycle where AI had not been used.

Currently, intra-uterine insemination (IUI) (see chapter 11, page 204) using a prepared pellet of sperm is being advocated by many units, alone or following ovarian stimulation with clomiphene citrate or gonadotrophins. However, controlled cycle data have led to the conclusion that compared with just having normal coitus, 37 cycles of IUI alone would have to be undertaken to get one additional pregnancy.

IUI in combination with ovulation induction agents appears to improve conception rates three-fold but controlled results are contradictory. Gonadotrophin plus IUI is more effective, with a mean 16% success rate compared with 6% for IUI plus clomiphene. The potential for serious complications from ovarian stimulation, such as multiple pregnancies and ovarian hyperstimulation syndrome, is, however, higher (see chapters 9 and 11, pages 128 and 207). Because of this, tertiary care centre facilities are needed for ovarian stimulation therapy.

Scientific placebo-controlled live-birth study data do not truly exist for IUI in this situation. Although IUI is advocated by many to be used before IVF itself, it is not free from complications. With such poor results it is doubtful that in the older patient, where time is at a premium, more than a maximum three cycles if any should be expended on such treatment pre IVF.

IVF and ICSI

Both IVF and ICSI are frequently employed in unexplained infertility. This is certainly valid provided they are not launched into immediately without a time-out interval being taken after the 'unexplained' label has been given. Both, but especially IVF, may also provide evidence as to cause, as the process of conception can be observed from initial sperm contact through to transfer, albeit in artificial in-vitro conditions.

There appears to be no advantage to ICSI over IVF in unexplained infertility and less can be learned about what may be going wrong in terms of sperm-egg penetration function than with IVF. Pregnancy rates per cycle are commensurate with those for other indications, at some 30%. However, a number of fertility units have noted outcome measures in this group of couples to be less favourable than for natural conceptions in terms of abortion, ectopic pregnancy, multiple pregnancy and take-home baby rates.

The results are considerably better than for any of the other active approaches on offer, but it must be noted that there is also a potentially positive placebo effect for being put on the waiting-list for IVF treatment or for conceiving immediately after a failed cycle. This is accepted to be up to about 16%. This placebo effect may also continue after IVF success. In the author's unit, 21% of those who had conceived with IVF achieved further success within two years without more therapy.

Gamete intra-fallopian transfer (GIFT)

Gamete intra-fallopian transfer (GIFT) has also been used, more in the past than today. This brings together extracted eggs and sperm outside the body, then transferring some of the mixture (up to two eggs per tube) back inside the woman. This, however, usually requires laparoscopy and, unlike IVF, has no diagnostic potential. Reported results are similar to IUI plus gonadotrophin stimulation (16%). However, doubt has been cast on the veracity of some of the data supporting this result.

Natural procreative technology (NaProTechnology)

Couples conventionally labelled as having 'unexplained infertility' seem to form the majority of the infertile patients undergoing NaProTechnology. This is why the technique has been described in this section, though such couples are moved by the NaProTechnology system practitioners from 'unexplained' into that of a known cause, frequently ovulatory in origin.

Not all health professionals involved in the field of infertility would agree with all of the basic premises underlying NaProTechnology, nor with how it is practised and the claims made for it. Doubts have been voiced as to the conclusions drawn from the data obtained, the diagnoses that are given to the patients and the drug regimes then sometimes used in individual cases. It is, however, certainly appropriate in a book such as this, designed primarily for infertile patients, to acknowledge that NaProTechnology exists and to try to explain its modus operandi for potentially interested parties.

It was developed in America at the Pope Paul VI Institute for Human Reproduction, Omaha. Practitioners state that it continues to evolve. There is now a network of centres in a number of countries. The term is used to describe a 'scientific, holistic process of investigation' of gynaecological problems, including infertility and recurrent miscarriage. It teaches couples to recognise, examine and record on 'Creighton Model Fertility Care System' charts the 'natural biological marker of fertility' of cervical mucus and its changes in quantity and quality from dry to peak and back during a menstrual cycle.

The followers of this technique state that looking closely at the patterns that emerge (usually over a three-month period) allows a thorough evaluation of the woman's 'fertility cycle'. It enables identification of abnormal menstrual and cervical mucus patterns and, by looking at oestradiol (E2) and progesterone (P) levels on ovulation peak day +7, subtle hormonal deficiencies can be found that could otherwise go undetected by routine hormonal tests.

Ovulatory levels of progesterone are set higher in this method by those involved than those considered to be usual in day 21 assays. It has been stated at presentations of the method that in some '80% of women thus tested, hormonal deficiencies on peak day +7 are found.' A scoring system has been devised. Deductions are made and a diagnosis of an underlying cause for the failure to conceive is then given and treatment prescribed, timed to the woman's cycle.

Depending on the diagnostic conclusions reached from the charts, treatment can include general and dietary advice, vitamin supplements, steroids, 'endorphin' therapy, ovarian hormonal stimulation, and hormone supplementation, often with 'natural progesterone'. The use of such drugs is on the premise that they are not being employed to help conception directly, but instead to get the woman to the point where cycles are 'normalised' and 'natural conception' is facilitated. The stated aim is to restore, usually within a three-month target period, normality to the appearance of the 'fertility care system chart' to show what are known as 'effective cycles' and thus optimise fertility potential for the couple.

To ensure the efficacy of this therapy, the charts are continued throughout the couple's time under the care of the practitioner. In the first three months, as part of the de-stress concept, attempts at conception are not encouraged as changes in therapy may need to be made. Ultrasound is used to ensure ovulation has occurred. If the woman is not pregnant after 12 effective cycles (this usually takes on average some 18-24 months to complete) further 'therapy' is not encouraged and the couple are 'counselled out'.

If not previously performed, laparoscopy is often recommended early on. Great store is set by the early diagnosis and treatment of endometriosis, which is thought to have a negative influence on the fertility cycle and increase miscarriage. In all this, the male is not ignored, and advice, usually as to lifestyle but sometimes the use of certain drugs, has been reported to help.

NaPro Technology, like much of infertility treatment, seems to suffer from a lack of properly designed placebo controlled trials. Correlations have been made between E2 and progesterone levels and different cervical mucus patterns at presentations of the method. The comparisons made with other therapies seem to be usually against IVF.

In a recent verbal report of 1239 NaProTechnology treatment cycles in 1072 couples, the cumulative live birth rate was found to be 25.5%. When this was adjusted for study drop-outs of almost 50%, the cumulative live birth rate rose to 52.8%. At what stage the drop-outs occurred was unclear, and what drugs were used and when was not stated.

Overall, these results appear to be commensurate with those expected from other approaches to the unexplained infertile couple, where data exist, including for IVF (the majority, however, also not controlled) and the known overall placebo rates that all investigations and treatments have in infertility (see chapter 5, pages 26-7), adjusted for age and length of infertility.

Personal Comment

Unless the investigations really do reveal a hitherto hidden cause, allowing the label 'unexplained infertility' to be replaced by something more concrete, the benefits of any therapy are likely to be no better than no treatment at all or a placebo (sugar) pill and yet have greater side-effects. All health professionals are likely to fall into the trap of prescribing treatment to couples labelled as having 'unexplained' or 'idiopathic' infertility at some time or other to satisfy either their own feelings of inadequacy or the patients' expectations of being given 'fertility drugs'. Couples need to understand that there is no placebo-controlled evidence for such treatment in unexplained infertility and that side-effects potentially outweigh any benefits.

In NaProTechnology, despite the claim that the intention is not to treat directly but to correct to normality an unexplained infertility situation so conception can then take place, drugs (often multiple) are very frequently employed. It is therefore not quite the natural system it is claimed to be. Whichever drugs are used, whatever the dosages, the same potential side-effects exist.

SECTION V: RECURRENT MISCARRIAGE (HABITUAL ABORTION)

Definition and background

Recurrent miscarriage is outside the strict definition of infertility. However, as many couples with this problem can remain childless despite conceiving and, in their eyes, are the same as infertile couples, it is appropriate to include the subject here.

Recurrent miscarriage is defined as three consecutive pregnancies, with the fetus under 500 grams, ending spontaneously before the 20th week of pregnancy. The incidence is 1% of women.

Causes

More than one factor may be present and the cause of individual miscarriages may not be the same each time. A cause may be specific to the male or the female or occur only when these two persons interact together. To avoid confusion, in this section, I will examine each possible cause as if it had the potential to be the sole causative factor. Categorisation into two groups helps. These are 'doubtful', where current data suggest a loose connection, and 'possible' where the association has more scientific validity but the final proof is lacking.

Doubtful

Severe acute infection
Any infection in the woman may cause miscarriage on a one-off basis if body temperature gets very high, especially if toxins are released or defence mechanisms are low.

Chronic infections
Many organisms have been blamed in the past. The list includes listeria, toxoplasmosis, brucella, mycoplasma, chlamydia, Herpes simplex and cytomegalovirus. However, many of these can normally be found in the vagina from time to time and whilst they can cause acute infection, in the absence of this, their chronic presence may have little or no effect on miscarriage. Hence, they are listed as doubtful.

Endocrine
Disorders such as underactive thyroid gland in the woman fall into this category, as do diabetes and polycystic ovarian syndrome.

Environmental
Exposure of either partner to certain herbicides, electromagnetic fields and radiation sources has been cited in the media as a cause of habitual miscarriage, but there are no sound scientific data to back this up. Alcohol, smoking and street drugs have also been similarly indicted both actively and passively.

Occupational hazards
Frequent exposure of women to anaesthetic gases, solvents, heavy

metals, VDUs, or industrial and agricultural chemicals has been cited in some studies and cleared in others. Currently our knowledge is inconclusive.

Possible

Genetic

Genetic factors in both male and female partners can sometimes play an important part in miscarriages. Sixty to seventy per cent of all miscarriage tissue has been found to be chromosomally abnormal. However, where there is a problem with recurrent spontaneous abortion, in only 3–5% of couples will there be an abnormal karyotype (arrangement of chromosomes).

There are many different types and causes of chromosomal abnormality. The majority are outside the intended scope of this book. The commonest abnormal chromosomal pattern to be concerned of here in respect to recurrent miscarriage is what is called a 'translocation'. This is where some of the chromosomal material in the cell following a breakage becomes interchanged between two or more different chromosomes and becomes sited in other than its usual places. If no overall loss of genetic material occurs this is known as a 'balanced translocation' and the person is a 'balanced translocation carrier'. This does not usually cause problems for the individual in terms of general health, although such types of abnormality are also increased in incidence in men with male factor infertility (see chapter 7, pages 43-4).

In this situation couples run the risk that some of their sperm and eggs may have an unbalanced chromosomal make-up (some genetic material is missing or excessive). If this sperm or egg rather than one featuring the balanced translocation is used in fertilisation then, even if the partner's gamete is normal, an unbalanced translocation is the result for the new embryo, leading to failure to implant or to miscarriage or to a child with mental or physical problems. This will recur with each unbalanced translocation created.

Genetic factors also encompass an inherited predilection for clotting (hereditary thrombophilias). Hypercoagulation conditions in women, such as Factor 5 Leiden mutation and antithrombin 111, have been strongly linked by many experts, but not by all, with recurrent miscarriage. There is a high likelihood of thrombosis (blood clot) formation in the placenta as pregnancy enhances the clotting response. This can lead to loss of utero placental function, which is the fetal lifeline, and miscarriage can occur.

Auto-immunity

Acquired autoimmune diseases in women such as systemic lupus erythematosis (SLE) can also be a possible cause of recurrent miscarriage due to an underlying clotting defect. Indeed, the presence of the lupus anticoagulant and/or anti-phospholipid antibodies and other anti-nuclear antibodies, even in the absence of clinical SLE, are important findings in someone who has suffered recurrent miscarriages in the second trimester, especially if anti-cardiolipin antibodies are also present (15% versus 2% in normal women). The pro-thrombotic (clotting) effect maybe on the development and subsequent functioning of the placenta.

Other antigens that the woman's immunological defence system perceives as foreign, thus leading to immunological incompatibility with either fetus or partner, have also been suggested as possible causes. These include natural killer T cells and shared parental human leucocyte antigens (HLA). However, to date, the lack of scientifically proven evidence suggests that testing and treatment for these factors should take place only in the context of properly designed scientific trials. There is not at present any specific immunological test that predicts the need for treatment.

Uterine

Some congenital anatomical defects of the uterus that distort its cavity (see Figure 6, page 66) may be associated with recurrent miscarriage as possibly can fibroids where the uterine shape is also distorted. Intrauterine adhesions (Asherman's syndrome) may also function similarly (see chapter 8, page 68).

Cervical incompetence
Cervical incompetence is a weakness in the circular muscle formation of the cervix. It may be congenital, or acquired by damage in a previous labour.

Metabolic
In itself, morbid obesity has been cited as a possible cause. A rare disorder of copper metabolism called Wilson's disease, which shows up in the coloured part of a woman's eyes, falls under this 'metabolic' heading.

Hormonal
'Hormone dysfunction in the woman' has traditionally been the most common explanation offered to couples. It is always linked to a possible deficiency in progesterone production, affecting the maintenance of very early pregnancy. It is a likely underlying cause but difficult to prove conclusively. It is one that remains to be suggested after all others have been excluded.

Diagnosis of cause

History

The couple's history can be very important in pointing towards a possible cause. Information is needed regarding past reproduction and especially the time of the losses: when they are early (4-6 weeks), this suggests a chromosomal abnormality; later (12+ weeks) a uterine or cervical problem. Past ultrasound findings may help also in diagnosing cause as would any results of cytogenetic analysis of previous conception products if such analysis had been performed.

Physical examination

Physical examination in the woman and man may be normal. Weight and body mass index (BMI) may be increased. This is unlikely to be a specific cause, but should enable discussion of lifestyle issue and the potential for anovulation and diabetes rather than as a likely possible specific cause.

A full examination of all systems (see chapter 6, pages 29-31) may reveal an underlying potentially significant disease. Fibroids may be felt abdominally and vaginally. Vaginal examination of the cervix may lead to a suspicion of cervical incompetence but it may take serial examinations during the next pregnancy to be more definite.

Specific investigations

Blood
Genetic
Tests should include peripheral blood 'karyotyping' (chromosomal screening) of both partners via the co-operation of a genetics laboratory. You should, however, be warned that tests may take some time for results to become available. They are expensive. Apparent normality does not always rule out a genetic cause. When positives are found, repeats and supplemental tests may be necessary to enable appropriate advice to be given by the clinical geneticist.

A screen for clotting factors, especially Factor 5 Leiden deficiency, may also be appropriate.

Auto-immune
In women, tests for SLE, antiphospholipid and anticardiolipin antibodies should be performed twice, at least six weeks apart.

Hormones
Serial progesterone levels in the luteal phase of the menstrual cycle and endometrial dating have both been used to try to show an underlying hormonal deficiency. However, replication in a subsequent cycle is dif-

ficult to prove, though that does not mean it may not be present.

NaProTechnology practitioners (see pages 179-82) believe endometriosis can 'add to the problem [of recurrent miscarriage] directly and by menstrual cycle hormonal influence'. They add in laparoscopy as a means of diagnosing and treating endometriosis in this situation.

Ultrasound, hysterosalpingogram and hysteroscopy

These can help to detect a congenital uterine abnormality, the latter two fairly exactly. However, ultrasound scans may help vaginal examinations where cervical incompetence is suspected.

Treatment and prognosis

No treatment

The theoretical risk of loss next time after three consecutive miscarriages is calculated to be some 40-45%. Where there has been one successful pregnancy first, the chance of success after three consecutive miscarriages is 55–60%. The chances of a pregnancy ending with a miscarriage increases with age, possibly due to a diminution in the quality of oocytes (eggs) or a possible increase in the chances of chromosomal abnormalities in the fetus. Following any miscarriage, even if the next conception is successful, there can be three times the normal risk of a low birth weight baby and a nearly 70% chance of a premature delivery.

Genetic

Where a specific chromosome abnormality is found in one of the couple, it may be found unwise or not possible to suggest any specific therapy towards conception using the gametes of that person. The help and advice of a clinical geneticist should be sought to determine any such prognosis before making a decision whether or not to go ahead as there are important implications for both the parents and the longed-for child.

Genetically caused miscarriage cases differ, as do the incidence, causes and types of chromosomal genetic abnormality or gene defect. In the case of a balanced translocation the chance of one being present in habitual miscarriage couples may be between 5-10%. Where a balanced translocation exists in one or other partner, as explained above (page 184), if the sperm or egg used has an unbalanced make-up, it will lead to an embryo having an unbalanced defective chromosomal make-up with genetic material becoming lost or excessive. However, not all the balanced translocator's gametes will be unbalanced and there is still likely to be an up to 40-50% chance of a healthy birth next time without any further intervention.

Utilising pre-implantation genetic diagnosis (PGD) as part of IVF for the next attempt at having a child may help resolve the dilemma. This can determine the sex of the embryo, which may be important in sex-linked disease, and possibly screen the embryos for the abnormality itself, after fertilisation but pre-implantation. This allows selection and transfer of only those embryos that are apparently normal (see page 224). Donor gametes can also be used to bypass the situation for the implicated partner (see page 197).

Where the problem is excessive blood clotting (hypercoaguability) due to a hereditary thrombophilia, low molecular-weight heparin therapy can be used during the pregnancy.

Immunological

Where anti-phospholipid or anti-cardiolipin antibodies are found, there seems to be benefit in utilising low-dose heparin and aspirin (see also chapter 8, page 73).

A controlled study has shown that in the presence of such antibodies some 10% may succeed without treatment, rising with heparin/aspirin therapy to some 70%. The aspirin is started with the diagnosis of pregnancy, and heparin injections are added in when the fetal heart becomes detectable. Both continue until late pregnancy, but the heparin also until six weeks after if there is a history of thrombosis.

So-called 'immunotherapies' such as injecting paternal lymphocytes, immunoglobulins or steroids into the female, have so far not borne out apparent early promise when subjected to scientific scrutiny. They are associated with significant hazards and considerable financial outlay. At present, no other such 'immunotherapy' can be justified as routine treatment. It should only be contemplated as part of a recognised registered independent ethically approved scientific study.

Uterine anatomical defects

Where uterine defects are considered significant and amenable to corrective surgery, they can be dealt with via an abdominal operative approach (utriculoplasty), or, if facilities and training permit, vaginally using an operating hysteroscope (see chapter 8, page 71-2). The aim is to try to restore anatomical normality as much as is possible (see Figure 6, page 66).

If significant uterine abnormalities can be corrected and there are no other factors, the chances of success next time should be as for the normal population, when the incidence of known miscarriage is approximately only 15-20%.

Cervical weakness/incompetence

The cervix can in theory be reinforced by putting a stitch around it via the vagina (cervical cerclage) in early pregnancy (after 12 weeks), removing it as late as possible (38 weeks). The encircling material can also be installed pre-pregnancy (occasionally during if early on and diagnosis of cause is sure) but this former requires a trans-abdominal approach.

Results are, however, controversial and have long been the subject of debate, possibly because of over-diagnosis of cervical incompetence in the past. Randomised trials have failed to demonstrate improved pregnancy outcome from the vaginal approach. Where there is irrefutable evidence of potential cervical weakness, the abdominal installation route may be the better way forward.

Hormones

A 'hormonal cause' is really the term used as an alternative to cause unknown. As previously stated, it is common practice to suggest there may be a menstrual cycle hormonal defect, especially in progesterone production. This is almost impossible to prove conclusively; the alternative used is to treat it empirically – that is, no truly proven reason for the treatment.

Circulating progesterone levels (see chapter 9, page 114) are not raised by progesterone supplements but high doses theoretically have the potential to give feminising side effects on a male embryo/fetus.

Human chorionic gonadotrophin injections (hCG) administered from first diagnosis of pregnancy have, however, been shown in a 'meta analysis' of all relevant studies to be somewhat better than placebo. hCG is what the body produces naturally to prolong the life of the corpus luteum (see page 109) from when pregnancy occurs until the placenta takes over the necessary hormone production. However, the diagnosis of hormone deficiency in these hCG studies was made by excluding other causes rather than on the basis of hormone levels. In two small ethically approved double-blind studies against placebo (neither myself as the doctor involved nor my patients knew whether they were getting active treatment or placebo), hCG had a success rate of between 83% and 100% versus 30-79% for placebo.

Ovulation induction, such as with clomiphene citrate and progestational luteal phase supplements, is sometimes used. This is really again a placebo-type of approach and likely therefore to have the usual 30% chance of success except in recurrent miscarriage patients with polycystic ovarian syndrome where it does seem to help.

NaProTechnology

In this section, it seems appropriate to draw attention to those advocating NaProTechnology for habitual miscarriage. The approach to habitual miscarriage reflects their approach to infertility (see pages 179-82) and starts in advance of the next conception. The underlying premise is the importance of achieving 'effective cycles', including the active laparoscopic management of endometriosis. Success in a recent small series of 15 such couples, reported to a meeting, was 77% for those who complied with their regime of therapy compared with 16% of those (number not cited) who started but then dropped out.

Tender loving care (TLC)

'TLC' is not doing nothing but is specifically directed at basic management of the next pregnancy, both prior to and as soon as possible when it occurs. The approach uses one-to-one consultations, supportive counselling and reassuring ultrasound scans (weekly at first) instead of empiric hormonal treatment if no cause is found.

Reports in couples who have had habitual miscarriage suggest excellent results with over 70% success in the next pregnancy compared with the generally accepted figures of 55-60%. This effect is very well worth noting, but in any case it should be the basic underlying norm for management in any habitual miscarriager's next pregnancy, even if active management is also being used.

Personal Comment

Recurrent miscarriage is very distressing. If this happens to you it is hard not to become obsessed by it. While some early miscarriages may sometimes be nature's way of getting rid of an abnormality this should not be allowed to create a background of fear for all subsequent conceptions.

Far better is to focus on the steps needed to find a cause and manage it. If none can be found, it is much better that you know.

Few specific therapies exist. If there may be an underly-

ing endocrine deficiency, what appears to work best empirically is hCG, the substance produced naturally to prolong the luteal phase of the menstrual cycle in very early pregnancy.

What certainly helps is TLC. You should expect this from the health care team to see you through these difficult times.

Chapter 11

Assisted Reproduction Techniques (ART)

MYTHS

1. AI results are as good as natural intercourse.
2. IVF cures all.

Assisted Reproduction – ART – is defined by the World Health Organisation (WHO) as including all treatments or procedures that involve the in-vitro (test tube) handling of human eggs (oocytes), sperm and embryos (in-vitro fertilisation or IVF/ICSI) for the purpose of establishing a pregnancy. However, artificial, or assisted, insemination (AI) is also included as an assisted reproductive technique by many countries, though not the USA.

The number of children born as a result of ART techniques as a percentage of all births is now becoming significant but varies from country to country. In the USA, for instance, it is 1% of total births, in the UK 1.6%, whereas in Denmark it has been reported as being some 4%.

SECTION I: ARTIFICIAL INSEMINATION (AI)

Definition and basic techniques

AI is defined as the deposition of male gametes (spermatozoa) into the female genital tract by means other than natural intercourse, with the purpose of achieving conception. It has been used in a DIY manner since time immemorial.

Sperm may be from a donor (AID) or the woman's husband or partner (AIH), but whatever the source of the sperm, there are a number of basic features that all AI procedures have in common.

Samples may be deposited, neat or following laboratory preparation, in the vagina, or the cervix, or the uterus (IUI) (see Figure 14, page 202). The aim is to perform the procedure in the peri-ovulatory phase of the menstrual cycle, one or two times within one cycle. A gap of one or two days can be allowed as sperm will live for some three days inside the woman.

Ovulation induction and formal follicle monitoring may or may not be used. Except for IUI, the insemination can be performed by the woman or her partner themselves (DIY AI), or under medical or paramedical supervision. A glass or plastic cannula (fine tube: see Figures 13 and 18, pages 200 and 228 respectively) can be used to insert the semen into the woman's vagina or cervix. She is best lying down for this and should rest for about 30 minutes afterwards.

Where IUI is utilised, the sperm sample needs to be prepared first by a washing method. Often, a simple culture medium is used. Culture media are fluids made up of a variety of compounds developed primarily to nourish and protect gametes and embryos during in-vitro procedures. Many different types exist, constructed for different situations.

In IUI washing the semen is necessary so as to avoid introducing infection from the seminal plasma (the liquid non-sperm part of semen) into the uterus. This may possibly also improve quality. A fine tube (catheter), containing the sample, is inserted through the cervical canal under direct vision, as provided by a speculum, and discharged into the lower part of the uterus.

Background to donor insemination (AID)

Historically, personal sourcing of semen is always likely to have taken place between friends and acquaintances (DIY), and still does. AID does not treat a male problem; it bypasses it.

Donor insemination as a specific medical procedure began in the UK in the 1930s and has been in widespread use for some 50 years, particularly since successful cryo-preservation (freezing) became available in the 1960s. Initially fresh semen was used but, precipitated by the advent of AIDS, almost universally donor sperm are now frozen at source and kept cryo-preserved in a sperm bank for a minimum of six months to clear the donor of disease before usage.

Rules about donor procreation vary widely from country to country. Some countries have controls on (UK) or guidelines for (USA) donors and the related procedures; others do not. Certainly, up until 2007, sperm-donor attempts at procreation were not allowed by law in Austria (except for one clinic) or Germany and only for IVF in Italy, Tunisia or Turkey. Specific registered banks are needed in France, Norway and Sweden. Donors must be known in the Netherlands, Norway, Sweden and the UK but anonymous in Singapore, Slovenia and Vietnam.

The supply of donors has become difficult and almost non-existent in countries where the traditional anonymity of the donor has been abolished such as the UK, Netherlands, Norway and Sweden. There can be religious constraints for some and limits on the number of offspring set by many, including six in Spain and ten in the UK.

Indications for AID

Male factor infertility

Male factor infertility has been the chief medical indication over the years. While intra-cytoplasmic sperm injection (ICSI; see pages 211-12) has transformed the prognosis for many such men, in the man who has no testes or whose testes are not functioning or who cannot ejaculate, AI with donor sperm may still need to be considered.

Genetic disease

Where the male partner has sex-linked genetic abnormalities that can be passed on to an offspring, AID with donor sperm is a way of bypassing the situation.

Infectious disease

Infectious diseases that make AID worthwhile at present include HIV positivity in the man, which could be life-threatening for his partner and/or the child if passed on. Using a non-infected donor bypasses this.

Severe Rhesus iso-immunisation

Where the mother has Rhesus negative blood and the father Rhesus positive, resulting in an immunological reaction that will damage the baby, the use of sperm from a Rhesus negative donor will again bypass the problem.

Female same-sex couples

Where women in a same-sex relationship desire pregnancy, AID can be the solution.

Checks before AID

Couples considering therapeutic AID via the clinic route need to satisfy themselves, before commencing, that AID is really acceptable to both partners and that there is a clear indication for it with no acceptable alternative. Significant thought needs to be given to the psycho-social issues;

donor therapy raises many potential legal, ethical, moral and social aspects that must be thought through and resolved before, rather than after, treatment has been started. These include parenthood certification, which differs from country to country, and the right to anonymity of parents and the donor versus the rights of the child to know its origins. Access to expert counselling can be very beneficial and many consider it to be essential.

In countries where there are no regulations, it is important that potential users find out as much as possible about the safeguards, donor recruitment policy, counselling and screening methods of the suppliers before a donor is accepted. Other information that needs to be ascertained includes: the availability of sperm from a specific donor and the possibility of obtaining a repeat after a previous success; the number of pregnancies per donor that are allowed; and the extent to which the clinic keeps records and for how long.

Details concerning the donor himself are needed, especially where a degree of matching is being attempted with regard, for example, to blood group, eye and skin colour and general interests. Using friends or relatives as donors can be problematic and is not to be encouraged; anonymous donors are preferred. Mixing in the partner's sperm, if some exist, is detrimental to the outcome as inter-reactions may occur that damage quality and outcome. Gamete or embryo mixing is not allowed in the UK. The woman needs to have a fertility evaluation first to ensure that she has no problems with conception that could make embarking on AID a waste of time.

AID cycle management

During treatment cycles, pinpointing the timing of ovulation before sperm insemination is particularly important. For women with regular 28-day cycles, no formal monitoring needs to be used at first (for up to three months) to prevent excessive stress. Home urine or saliva kits that pinpoint the periovular phase may be useful as detailed previously in chapter 9 on ovulation (page 116); as used in IVF, vaginal ultrasound tracking of follicle development is the best of the formal methods.

As with IVF (see page 218-9), injections of hCG will promote and help to time (34 hours later) the rupture of a mature follicle to produce an egg. The anti-oestrogen ovarian stimulant, clomiphene citrate, may be used (see chapter 9, page 123), even if the woman is apparently ovulating initially, as the stress of the situation may cause this to stop. Gonadotrophins are rarely necessary and, where they are, IVF with the donor sperm may be preferable. It is more controllable.

Some couples prefer to collect the semen from the bank, transport it home frozen and perform the insemination post-thaw (into the vagina or cervix, but not the uterus) in the privacy of their own home (DIY AID). They may find it less stressful. Transport facilities that help keep the sperm frozen until use are a possibility but, unlike in the clinic, it is not possible to check that the sperm quality is satisfactory after thawing before use at home. A little time at room temperature is needed before insemination to ensure the sperm have recovered from the freezing process.

IUI AID is seldom indicated but may come into play if other insemination routes are not possible or fail. It needs hospital intervention as in IUI AIH (see below).

Whether at home or in the clinic, the sperm are contained in a straw or in a small screw-top ampule (jar) before insemination. The specimen is unfrozen (10 minutes at room temperature) and put into a sterile syringe (generally 1-10 millilitre capacity) for insemination into the vagina or cervix depending upon choice. Treatment length varies. Six to an absolute maximum of 12 cycles is recommended.

If ovulation can be pinpointed with a degree of certainty, it seems to make little difference to the outcome whether one or two inseminations are used per cycle. Some published reports have found double inseminations per cycle giving better results, but others have found this no better than single.

Where the IUI route is used, the procedure is exactly the same as for AIH IUI (see pages 205-6).

Figure 13 Basic types of insemination equipment

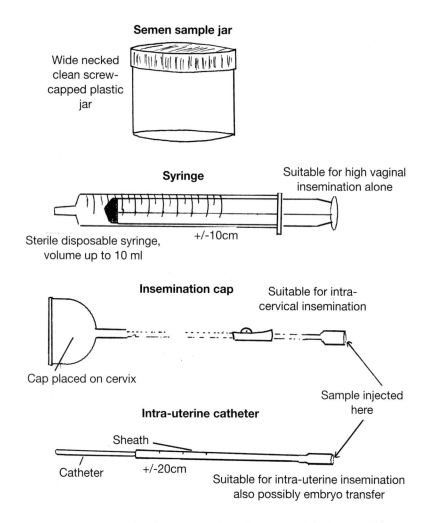

Semen sample jar

Wide necked clean screw-capped plastic jar

Syringe

Suitable for high vaginal insemination alone

Sterile disposable syringe, volume up to 10 ml

+/-10cm

Insemination cap

Suitable for intra-cervical insemination

Cap placed on cervix

Sample injected here

Intra-uterine catheter

Sheath

Catheter

+/-20cm

Suitable for intra-uterine insemination also possibly embryo transfer

Note: Illustrations of equipment are generic and do not illustrate any particular manufactured type. They are also not drawn to scale.

AID prognosis

If the couple is properly selected and the woman is in good health, cycle fecundity rates using AID with fresh semen can be expected to be on a par with natural conception, whatever the site of insemination, if all other factors including female age are equal (see page 9). However, because of the use of frozen semen, this figure has now dropped by some 15-25%, and the time to conception has doubled. French national figures give a pregnancy rate of 10.3% per unstimulated cycle in up to six cycles. Monthly fecundability rises with the number of cycles performed but drops as time goes on. One UK study gave a cumulative conception rate after six months of 48%, rising slowly to 66% after 12.

Clinics no longer use the full sample; it is divided into 'aliquots' (portions) for freezing. Freezing in itself has some effect on the quality and life of sperm. Cycle stimulation appears to make little difference to the pregnancy rate from such AID (live births per single unstimulated cycle are 9.1% versus 10.3% for stimulated) but there is increased risk of multiple pregnancy with the latter.

IUI seems to have some advantage over intra-cervical deposition, though only when frozen semen is used. For male factor infertility, IUI AID is still likely to be less effective than ICSI; for ICSI the European Society of Human Reproduction and Embryology (ESHRE 2004 in *Human Reproduction* 2008; 23: 756-771) gives a pregnancy rate of 18.7% under and 8.4% over 40 compared with 29.8% per transfer for ICSI. To have your own genetic child if possible is invariably felt to be preferable.

There are psycho-social issues to contemplate when reviewing the prognosis of AID, remembering that the wellbeing of the child is paramount. It remains to be seen whether disclosure of the child's origin leads to a greater chance of psychological disturbance as he or she grows up, akin to that sometimes seen in adoption. Indubitably, difficulties will always exist in AID, increased by the clandestine nature of many such conceptions. Long-term effects have rarely been researched but seem to show that few couples regret what they have done.

Figure 14 Potential sites for insemination

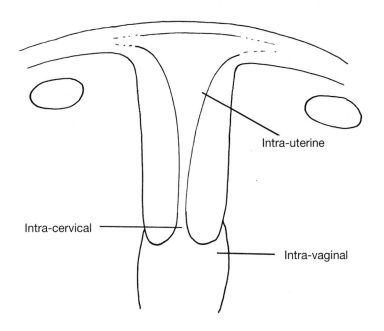

Indications for partner insemination (AIH)

Male sub-fertility

Over the years AIH ('H' used to signify husband) has been used when poor quality sperm are being produced. However, not surprisingly, results have always been disappointing. With the advent of ICSI (intra-cytoplasmic sperm injection), this use of AIH has fallen (see page 57).

Anatomical abnormalities

The main justifiable medical indication for AIH is when deposition of sperm of normal quality into the vagina is being physically prevented. Such situations are rare and include, in the man, congenital or acquired penile deformities and retrograde ejaculation (see chapter 7, pages 57-

8). In the woman, there may be vaginal or cervical strictures or blockages (see chapter 10, page 139). Specimens obtained by penile vibrators or electro-ejaculation from men with spinal injuries or neurological illness preventing coitus also come into this category. While DIY AIH can be used in these situations, such semen specimens are frequently small or of poor quality and may need to be quality checked before insemination, especially if they are not being obtained at sufficiently frequent intervals. IUI can be used in an attempt to improve matters. However, ICSI, using what is obtained by such ejaculatory methods or via testicular biopsy, may be a better bet.

Erectile dysfunction

Where there are collectable nocturnal emissions or there is intractable premature ejaculation, DIY AI with vaginal or cervical deposition is particularly suitable.

Semen frozen and banked for medical reasons

Semen cryo-preservation can be offered to men with cancer and other diseases, in an attempt to preserve their ability to have children, where the necessary therapy might render them sterile. Where multiple specimens of good quality have been preserved, AIH may be used, at any of the three sites, by the clinic or DIY, to attempt conception rather than trying ICSI. Vasectomy is not usually a medical indication for banking sperm.

'Anti-sperm antibody' presence

For those who believe 'anti-sperm antibodies' (see chapter 10, page 142) are a treatable cause of infertility, IUI can be used. It is hoped that washing will get rid of the antibodies detected by the tests on the surface of the sperm. If the quality of the post-washing specimen is poor, then ICSI is preferable from the start.

'Cervical factor'

Where the post-coital test (PCT) is continually negative (chapter 10) but the man has a normal sperm count it may be worth considering IUI if infertility persists and no other possible cause can be detected (see placebo effect, chapter 5, pages 26-7 and chapter 10, page 143).

Unexplained infertility

For 'unexplained infertility', where the semen parameters are within normal limits, AI is an empirical therapy (there is no scientific evidence for its use). Nevertheless, this is now the main 'indication' for AI usage by the IUI route, both with and without ovulation induction. Unless the semen specimen does not wash well, some units insist on a minimum of three cycles of IUI before going through to IVF.

Poor response to ovarian stimulation in an IVF cycle

IVF may require ovarian stimulation with drugs. Where there is a poor ovarian response to this with, say, only a single follicle produced, some fertility units convert the IVF cycle to IUI rather than stopping the cycle altogether.

Managing AIH treatment cycles

General

AIH has considerably less potential to cause psycho-social issues than AID. However, couples need to think about the choice between AIH and other alternatives before embarking on the process, especially if time is of the essence because of the woman's age. There are the same practical issues as for AID – the need to target peri-ovulation, the monitoring methods, and, especially, the precautions where ovulation stimulation is used to avoid hyperstimulation and multiple pregnancies (see also chapter 9, page 128, and pages 234 and 236 in this chapter).

Vaginal and cervical routes

DIY AIH may be more acceptable to the couple and can easily be arranged where good quality whole fresh semen samples are the initial source. The specimen can be checked to see if it is normal in advance but the vaginal or cervical route will need to be chosen. Home kits for testing ovulation may help with timing (see chapter 9, page 116) but unlike the hospital setting this may not be quite as important. The opportunity for multiple attempts is not constrained; you can do it when you fancy and privacy, intimacy and sexuality can be preserved. Instruction on technique is needed and a PCT-like check after the first attempt is wise if possible.

Best collection practices to aim for are: abstaining from ejaculation for two to three days; collection into a wide-necked sterile sterylene vessel (plastic-like jar); transfer into a sterile syringe (up to 10 millilitres capacity usually) for insemination into the chosen area of the female genital tract (see Figures 13 and 14, pages 200 and 202). Whether the fresh sample has been obtained by masturbation or otherwise, it should always be protected at body temperature to prevent the cold killing off the sperm if transfer into the syringe and insemination are not to be immediate, or if the sample is being brought into the clinic (it needs to arrive within two hours of production) for the insemination to be carried out there. Putting the screw-topped jar in an internal jacket pocket or transporting it down the woman's cleavage are both good options in this regard.

Intra uterine insemination (IUI)

Intra uterine insemination (IUI) is invariably carried out in the clinic. The woman's cycle, either natural or more often stimulated (with clomiphene citrate or more rarely with gonadotrophins), is monitored and the likely timing of the next peri-ovular phase determined. An appointment is then made for an IUI attempt.

This involves the man producing his semen sample and this being quality tested by the clinic. As I have said earlier, if the neat sample is used infection may be introduced or there may be chemical/allergic reaction and excess volume can cause uterine spasm. For this reason, the sample, if deemed suitable, is washed in a sterile medium and a portion of it containing between 5- and 20-million sperm in 0.5 millilitres is prepared by the laboratory for insemination. Similarly to an embryo transfer, the fluid is then injected slowly via a fine catheter inserted through the cervix directly into the lower part of the uterus under direct speculum vision (see Figure 18, page 228). The woman rests up for a while (up to 10 minutes) and then departs to resume normal life.

The process is often repeated a second time during the same peri-ovular phase. It is usual to try this approach for between three and six cycles and in some units it is almost mandatory to try for at least three cycles in couples with so-called 'unexplained infertility' before IVF is considered.

AIH prognosis

Where the semen sample is adequate

Where semen samples are of good quality, normal pregnancy rates have been noted anecdotally with DIY AI in couples with anatomical coital difficulties and with psycho-sexual problems. In unexplained infertility, by definition, semen is of good quality. When IUI is used, prognosis is tempered by the woman's age and length of infertility. There are few national registries giving annual success rates. Overall results are controversial and published figures range from 5% to 70% per patient. IUI alone does not appear to enhance pregnancy rates over an expected placebo effect but, when used with ovarian stimulation, prognosis does seem to be a little nearer that for IVF (30%) when cumulative conception and delivery rate results are calculated (taking into account pregnancies achieved within a timescale of a number of consecutive treatment cycles). No data anywhere, however, give results consistently above 15% per cycle. Not all publications agree, but the majority of randomised studies seem to show that double IUI attempts per cycle do slightly enhance the chances of pregnancy over single (12.5% versus 8.3%).

The case for using gonadotrophins is stronger, giving an 18% pregnancy rate per cycle compared with clomiphene citrate (11%) or timed intercourse (4.5%); but, as is clearly shown in discussions elsewhere (chapter 9, page 128 and this chapter, pages 234 and 236), using gonadotrophins can be much more problematic.

The latest figures for ART published by the European Society of Human Reproduction and Embryology (ESHRE 2004 in *Human Reproduction* 2008; 23(4): 756-771) come from 19 countries and record all IUI AIH attempts. These show an overall clinical pregnancy rate of 12.6% in women under 40 years of age and of 8.2% in 15 of these countries if they are over that. Details of what ovarian stimulation practices were used and the number of active follicles were not given in this report but it is highly likely stimulation was used in the vast majority of women as, in those who were under 40, 11.9% of the subsequent deliveries were twins and 1.3% were triplets.

Where the semen sample is already poor

Where the semen sample is already poor, vaginal or cervical deposition is unlikely to succeed, whether using DIY or ART unit-based therapy, and ICSI maybe advisable from the start, especially if the semen does not wash well and the sperm die prematurely. In the latter case, the same can be said for IUI. However, although IUI results (4-5%) appear better than those for timed intercourse (2.4%) or intracervical deposition (2%) if the specimen washes well, even with ovarian stimulation they are no better than 4-6%. Experience does, however, seem to differ from unit to unit. It therefore appears wise for each to set up its own criteria for IUI treatment in these circumstances. You should enquire as to what these are and on what results they are based.

Spinal injury patients are a problem in that often the first few samples obtained are poor. Quality of semen may improve if treatment is persisted with. Additionally, general anaesthetic may be needed because pain and high blood pressure may occur with electro-ejaculation, though not with vibrators. Testicular biopsy and ICSI may be a better option here (page 212).

Where semen has been frozen pre-treatment

The hope and opportunity to procreate that cryo-preserving sperm can give the sick individual is immeasurably positive psychologically. The illness may affect sperm quality and hence freezability so ICSI may be necessary. However, if pre- and post-thaw quality is good, there is no reason why (all other parameters affecting fecundity being equal) live birth results should not be similar to those from AID banks of some 10% per cycle. When the sick person has recovered and procreation is eventually attempted, in many cases semen production will be found to have recovered and the cryo-preserved specimens can be discarded.

Personal Comment

AI is not for everyone. Embarking on any donor therapy (sperm or egg) needs prior in-depth thought, professional advice and counselling from someone experienced in the area. Sperm donor insemination can be remarkably successful and with appropriate attention to selection, no child is likely to be thought of as not truly the couple's. After all, the maternal side is still making its normal contribution to pregnancy and to the baby's looks. Secrecy or disclosure about the means of conception is still a dilemma. This is, I feel, very understandable but if the former course is chosen do not forget that secrets often seem to come out at an inappropriate time no matter what precautions are taken. Where the latter option is chosen, support is again needed with advice as to how and when will be best to disclose.

Semen freezing to preserve procreational ability should be on offer as part of treatment for male cancer and other relevant diseases, with ICSI available in the background when samples are poor.

In a long-standing unexplained infertility situation where, due to age, time is of the essence, to delay IVF and be pressured into having IUI plus superovulation first for three to six cycles is, I feel, very hard to justify on moral never mind cost-effective grounds, especially in the older woman. While it has been calculated that IVF is approximately twice as costly per live birth as IUI, take-home baby rates per cycle are almost invariably at least double.

SECTION II: IN VITRO FERTILISATION (IVF)

Definitions and background

IVF has been defined by the WHO as an Assisted Reproductive Technology (ART) procedure involving extra-corporeal (outside the body) fertilisation. Although the offspring of the procedure are commonly called 'test tube babies' and the eggs are initially collected into such a receptacle (see Figures 15 and 17, pages 210 and 220), the procedure actually involves fertilisation outside the body in a laboratory petri dish ('in vitro' means literally 'in glass').

The fertilised egg(s) or zygote/ embryo(s) then grow(s) in the dish in an incubator until deemed mature for transfer (between days 2 and 5, see Figure 16, page 218). It/they are transferred to the uterus via the cervix using a syringe and cannula (see Figure 18, page 228). For pregnancy to be established, an embryo must successfully achieve implantation in the wall of the uterus (see chapter 2) and continue to grow.

Modifications in methodology have led to many acronyms for this group of procedures. The commonest term used – in vitro fertilisation (IVF) – really encompasses all. In common use also is 'ICSI' – that is, intra cytoplasmic sperm injection. ICSI differs from IVF in only one particular. Instead of placing prepared sperm next to the egg so that natural penetration and fertilisation of the egg can occur, in ICSI, a

Figure 15 Schematic diagrams of IVF and ICSI

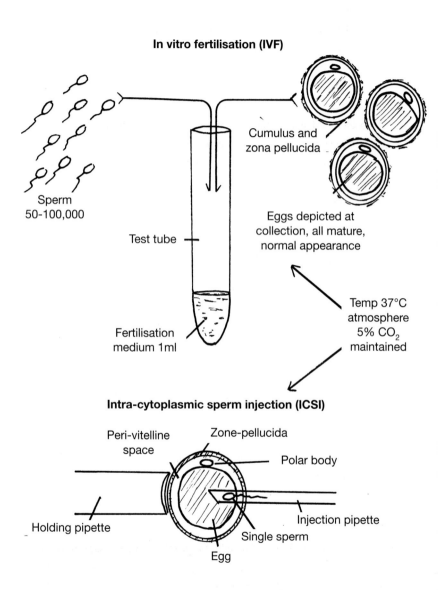

In vitro fertilisation (IVF)

Cumulus and
zona pellucida

Sperm
50-100,000

Test tube

Eggs depicted at
collection, all mature,
normal appearance

Temp 37°C
atmosphere
5% CO_2
maintained

Fertilisation
medium 1ml

Intra-cytoplasmic sperm injection (ICSI)

Peri-vitelline
space

Zone-pellucida

Polar body

Holding pipette

Injection pipette

Single sperm

Egg

Note: Gametes and
apparatus not to scale

single motile sperm is injected directly into the egg, or oocyte, (one per egg) to attempt fertilisation.

The first success with IVF was reported in 1978, and with ICSI in 1992. Today, Costa Rica excepted, both procedures are used worldwide. How they are controlled varies hugely, from legislation with or without a licensing body, to guidelines to be followed voluntarily, through to no rules at all except what the individual clinic may lay down.

Also included within the definition of ART is gamete intra fallopian tube transport (GIFT). In this procedure eggs are retrieved, sperm added and the mixture returned to the fallopian tubes (usually with two eggs per tube) for fertilisation to take place. It is not performed so often nowadays (see pages 178-9).

Indications for IVF/ICSI

Tubal factor

The first attempts at IVF were directed at by-passing tubal-factor problems as tubal surgery had shown such poor prognosis. However, microsurgery (see chapter 8, page 86) has improved results and if it is available, and appropriate to the situation, it should be attempted first.

Tubal damage is one of the main indications for IVF and may account for up to one third of cases in most parts of the world. Severe endometriosis (see chapter 8, page 102) affecting the tubo-ovarian pickup mechanism (the mechanism by which eggs enter the fallopian tubes) is also a significant indication.

Male factor

Initial attempts to use IVF for male factor problems were disappointing. The worse the quality of the semen, the poorer the success rates. This led to attempts to place the sperm next to the egg (sub zonal, or SUZI) and then to inject a sperm into the egg (ICSI). This latter is now the treatment of choice in this situation.

ICSI was first used with poor quality ejaculated sperm. This continues to be the case but indications now may also include sperm antibody problems and azoopermia, where sperm can be extracted from men who are apparently producing no sperm at ejaculation. This may be because of outflow obstruction or where testicular function is minimal but some sperm production is going on; as long as there is any production, it may be possible to obtain sperm by epididymal aspiration (PESA) or from the testis by removing some cells via a needle (biopsy) or taking a piece (TESA, see page 53).

About one third of couples who are considered for ART fit the category of truly needing ICSI. However, in some parts of the world, ICSI has almost totally replaced IVF as fertilisation rates are thought to be higher. There are, however, potential problems with offspring from ICSI, who may have a higher incidence of some congenital abnormalities. Pregnancy results are almost the same leading the USA government through its Centers for Disease Control and Prevention (CDC http://www.cdc.gov/art) to consider both together when reporting annual results.

Unexplained infertility

Couples labelled as having 'unexplained infertility' also account for about one third of ART cases, using it either as primary therapy or after empirical treatment (see chapter 10, pages 176-80) has failed.

Ovulation problems

Ovulation problems are a rare indication for IVF, but IVF can be considered after long-term failure to conceive despite ovulation being induced successfully. In addition, if an excessive number of ovarian follicles (above three: see chapter 9, pages 124-5) are produced in a cycle stimulated by gonadotrophins where in vivo conception is the aim, rather than cancelling the cycle it can in some circumstances be converted to an IVF cycle instead provided the couple concerned have been well counselled about the risks and benefits and given time to consider and sign an informed consent form.

Where the woman's ovaries have failed completely, donor eggs have to be utilised and IVF is the only option (pregnancy rate per donation 35.6%, ESHRE 2004).

Genetic problems

Where a detectable or sex-linked congenital abnormality is a possibility, pre-implantantion genetic diagnosis (PGD) can be employed in some countries. A cell, or blastomere, can be extracted from a day 2-3 IVF embryo for analysis. This enables selection of the appropriate sex or of unaffected embryos for transfer (see also phase 3 of treatment below, pages 224-5).

Before acceptance for a treatment cycle

Consent

If IVF is deemed a suitable treatment, before commencing on a cycle you will be asked to give your 'informed consent' to the treatment as a whole, and maybe also to some specific stages when these are variations from the norm. Expect to be supplied early on in your visits with written and verbal information and copies of the consent forms.

Physicians usually conduct the signing of these but before signing it can be invaluable to talk to other staff and also to make use of formal counselling sessions, which in some jurisdictions or clinics may be compulsory.

Information giving and receiving

There should be ample time for discussion with clinic staff about the programme and clinic policies, the implications and responsibilities on both sides, the potential problems and the potential prognosis for the particular couple. This is the best way of confirming that you as a couple are suitable or of detecting problems that may need to be addressed successfully first for you to be included for IVF.

Such exclusion criteria vary according to the clinic and/or the regulatory body concerned; they may include drug/chemical dependency, couple disharmony or ambivalence, and morbid obesity. Direct and hidden cost implications also need to be understood (see pages 18-19).

Preliminary work-up

The preliminary work-up may well differ from clinic to clinic. In most, the feeling is that a full fertility profile should have been completed to ensure there is a valid indication for IVF. In the IVF clinic itself, in-depth semen analysis should be performed and the response to the semen preparational methods tested before fertilisation is attempted.

If it is possible that semen may not be available at egg collection, some should be cryopreserved before treatment in the woman is started (see pages 154 and 229).

Hormone levels in the woman (FSH, LH, E2) are often estimated on day 3 of the cycle. This has been found useful in helping to determine the woman's ovarian reserve (having sufficient eggs left in her ovaries to enable her to be able to develop a number of follicles at the same time when the ovaries are artificially stimulated). If it is high (FSH 15+ IU/l), then response to ovulation stimulation may be so poor as to make an IVF attempt inappropriate. Other measures of this, none of which is perfect either (see chapter 9, page 122), include early-in-the-cycle counts of early (antral) follicles, inhibin B and anti-Mullerian hormone levels in blood or the clomiphene challenge test (see page 119).

General wellbeing is usually checked in advance, including weight and BMI, rubella status and cervical smear normality. Women are urged to start taking folic acid supplements and vitamin B_{12} if not already on them. A maximum of 4 units of alcohol per week should be the rule for the woman. The clinic will need to know the viral status of both partners, usually assessing HIV, hepatitis B and C status at the very least. Other clinics may also screen for syphilis, chlamydia and cytomegalovirus (CMV). Where any tests are positive, further action may be needed. Referral to a unit with appropriate facilities for treatment is recommended.

Where the indication for ICSI is oligozoospermia (very low sperm density of under five million), down to men with azoospermia, it is essential for the man to be tested for genetic karyotype (the number and structure of chromosomes he has) as there is an increased incidence of genetic abnormalities in such men due to the possibility of an abnormal chromosomal pattern. Chromosome abnormalities may be found in some 3-4% of ICSI candidates with Y male chromosome deletions (a loss of DNA that results in a part of that gene or even a part of a chromosome being missing) in 2%. In my clinic, the abnormal karyotype incidence increased to some 7.3% in azoospermic men. Where there is congenital absence of the vas deferens (see Figure 4, page 38) causing azoospermia, testing for cystic fibrosis (CF) gene deletions gives up to 70% positives even when all the men were healthy and not clinically CF sufferers.

The treatment cycle

Starting

Following agreement by all parties and informed consent forms being signed by both partners, the couple will be made ready to start the programme. The timing of this may depend on availability of a slot in some clinics and in others it will be down to the couple's own preferences and to menstrual cycle dates.

Types of IVF

IVF may be attempted using immature eggs (oocytes) that are allowed to mature in vitro, but this approach is still under research scrutiny. The latest published 2004 ESHRE data show a pregnancy rate of 10% from 109 cycles in two countries using IVM. However, in general clinical IVF the target oocyte will be a mature (metaphase 2) egg.

Mature oocytes can be obtained via a natural cycle without drugs or via a 'modified natural cycle', where drugs such as human chorionic gonadotropin (hCG) are given when the follicle is ripe, or an aromatase inhibitor (see chapter 9, page 132) is used to stimulate the ovary, but the aim is to collect only one oocyte. A 'mild IVF cycle' can also be used such as where lesser dosages of gonadotropin are given in combination with a GnRH antagonist, but the aim will then be to collect more than one egg (between two and seven).

Conventional IVF

While this latter approach may be the future for IVF, at present the vast majority of IVF cycles still use what is termed 'conventional IVF' methodology. The in-depth details of the procedure (see algorithm, figure 16, page 218) are described here and form the basis of the rest of the chapter.

Differences may occur from clinic to clinic in some details of day-to-day management and these may be a reflection of the regulations the clinic is working under. In fresh cycles, differing types of drugs, dosages and monitoring maybe utilised. Analgesia for egg collection may differ. The laboratory may use different culture media. The number, timing and method of embryo transfer and luteal support may also not always be the same. The underlying basics will, however, be the same. I will describe those still most commonly used noting only major differences where these reflect a growing alternative practice that might become the norm at a future date.

Phase One – Ovarian stimulation

Down regulation

Initial attempts at IVF used women's own natural cycles. However, results were found to be better if more eggs could be collected following ovarian stimulation. Gonadotropins and clomiphene citrate were originally used for ovarian stimulation. However, cycle control was poor and there were difficulties with timing egg collection. To counter this a treatment regime called 'down regulation' was introduced (see chapter 9, page 125).

Following a baseline ultrasound (US) scan of the ovaries, and also sometimes a test for blood oestradiol (E2), a gonadotrophin releasing hormone agonist (GnRHa) is given by injection or nasal spray in a number of daily doses, initially for two weeks, starting on day 1 of the menstrual cycle or mid-luteal phase. This stops the woman's own gonadotrophin FSH from being produced and interfering with the gonadotrophin that will be given. As a result, the woman's response to ovarian stimulation is somewhat more predictable.

At the end of the two-week period, if the ovaries are inactive (down-regulated), ovarian gonadotrophin drug stimulation starts. The GnRHa treatment is continued alongside this until the ovarian follicles are ripe.

In some centres, a gonadotrophin releasing hormone antagonist is now being used instead of the agonist, but as yet this is not widespread. This latter approach aims to produce the same result and ovarian control, but with less stimulation and hopefully therefore fewer side effects. The antagonist is used during ovarian gonadotrophin stimulation itself rather than prior to it.

Gonadotrophins

The aim of ovarian stimulation is to promote the formation and persistence of a number of follicles – ideally six to eight. Gonadotrophins are used for this; the present choice for injection is usually between manufactured recombinant follicular stimulating hormone (rFSH) and FSH extracted from menopausal urine (uFSH). This latter often contains either 'purified' FSH or FSH plus hCG (see chapter 9, pages 124-5). Each has its merits but results are similar whatever is used.

Starter dosage can be pragmatic (the same for all), or differ based on factors such as age or potential ovarian reserve. The presence of factors that may make the response excessive, such as PCOs and be-

Figure 16 Algorithm of a non-complicated down-regulated IV cycle

Note: Some clinic-specific
   variations may occur

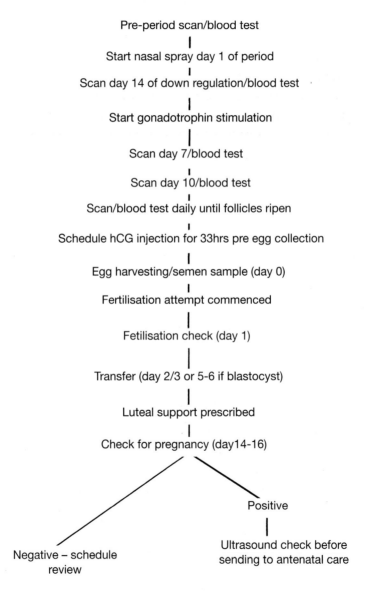

Pre-period scan/blood test

Start nasal spray day 1 of period

Scan day 14 of down regulation/blood test

Start gonadotrophin stimulation

Scan day 7/blood test

Scan day 10/blood test

Scan/blood test daily until follicles ripen

Schedule hCG injection for 33hrs pre egg collection

Egg harvesting/semen sample (day 0)

Fertilisation attempt commenced

Fetilisation check (day 1)

Transfer (day 2/3 or 5-6 if blastocyst)

Luteal support prescribed

Check for pregnancy (day14-16)

Positive

Negative – schedule
review

Ultrasound check before
sending to antenatal care

ing underweight, may lead to lesser starter doses to try to forstall ovarian hyperstimulation occurring. Whatever dosage is chosen, the response cannot ever be predicted exactly. Often the woman herself or her partner administers the injection daily after being shown how. The route is sub-cutaneously for rFSH; for uFSH it is sub-cutaneously or intra-muscularly.

In most units the same initial dosage is given for the first five to seven days, after which progress to date can be determined by monitoring ultrasound ovarian follicle number and size plus or minus oestradiol levels. If the results are satisfactory, the regimen and monitoring can be continued until the majority of the follicles are ripe enough (18-19 mm diameter on ultrasound) for the woman to be ready for egg collection. The gonadotrophin injections and GnRHa are then stopped.

hCG or sometimes, but more rarely, recombinant (rLH) is then prescribed to mature the follicles further and simulate the normal body LH surge (see chapter 9, page 124). A GnRHa can be used instead in an antagonist cycle (see page 217). This enables the timing of the egg collection to be arranged for some 33-35 hours later. Close monitoring is important.

Some units monitor only twice, at the start and at a fixed end point, using the same dosages throughout until hCG is given; others see the woman more frequently (six or so times) during ovarian stimulation.

Phase Two – Oocyte retrieval

Laparoscopy was used to give direct access to the ovaries in the past, but egg harvesting is nowadays attempted via the vagina under ultrasound guidance. Pain relief is usually provided but can vary from nothing, to employing a sedative such as Diazepam, to using a potent analgesic agent like pethidine, through to formal sedo-analgesia using a midazalam/fentanil mix administered by an anaesthetist.

A specially shaped vaginal ultrasound probe with a long needle attached visualises the ovarian follicles (see Figure 17, overleaf). The needle pierces the vaginal wall, enters each follicle in turn and aspirates it

Figure 17 Generic drawing of a vaginal probe and egg collection apparatus

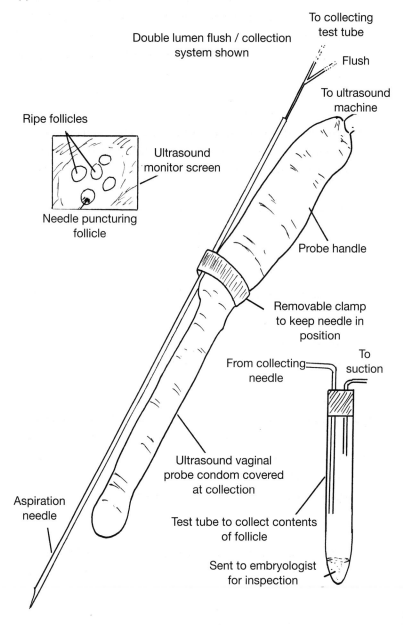

To collecting test tube

Double lumen flush / collection system shown

Flush

To ultrasound machine

Ripe follicles

Ultrasound monitor screen

Needle puncturing follicle

Probe handle

Removable clamp to keep needle in position

From collecting needle

To suction

Ultrasound vaginal probe condom covered at collection

Aspiration needle

Test tube to collect contents of follicle

Sent to embryologist for inspection

(sucks out the contents). Hopefully, immediate examination of the fluid by an embryologist will confirm the presence of an egg; the process can then be repeated until all follicles have been emptied. Formal flushing (cleansing out by injecting fluid) of follicles is used in many units if aspiration alone fails. Where there is a possibility of infection or of endometriosis developing, prophylactic antibiotic cover should be used.

While egg collection is progressing, the male partner will be asked to produce a semen sample, usually on site, unless cryo-preserved sperm are to be used. This sample is handed into the laboratory for processing.

Following completion of egg collection and a period of recovery in the clinic (30 minutes) the woman is usually free to leave, if deemed well enough, accompanied by her partner, to rest for up to 24 hours. She should not be alone or drive. The couple then keep in touch with the clinic on a daily basis, learning how fertilisation is progressing and working to the date for possible transfer.

Potential complications during phases one and two of a treatment cycle

An allergic reaction
An allergic reaction can occur with any drug administration.

Poor down regulation
If down regulation has not been achieved by day 14, the GnRHa can be doubled and continued for a further week before abandoning the cycle if this does not work. Down regulation can give rise to the formation of ovarian cysts in up to 10% of women. Such a cyst may need to be aspirated via the vagina if over 5 cm, endometriotic or in the way, before continuing.

Ovarian response is abnormal
When the ovarian response is poor, the choice is between increasing the dosage or stopping and restarting a new cycle with a higher gonadotrophin dose. In my clinic (reported in *Rotunda Hospital HARI Clinical Report* 2004) cancellations were 11%: CDC USA reported 12% in 2004.

Reactions can, however, differ on sequential cycles and even with increased dose of drugs may be no better. They are dependent on age and ovarian reserve. Reviewing possible causes, cancelling, and then trying again appears to work better than increasing the dosage at the time.

Chronic poor responders are the subject of much debate and empirical therapy. Their only option may be to consider using donor eggs.

If the response is considered excessive and many follicles are produced, there can be real danger, particularly of OHSS (ovarian hyperstimulation syndrome) as described below (also chapter 9, page 125). The choice is between cutting the dosage and reviewing daily, coasting (stopping gonadotrophin therapy), or abandoning the cycle, giving no hCG and banning coitus. If you and your doctors decide to carry on, it is worth considering freezing all resulting embryos.

Complications of egg collection

The procedure can be very painful, depending on the type of analgesia used (see also chapter 12, page 249). There can also be haemorrhage or bowel perforation (this maybe unrecognised and can be self-sealing). Some pain (period-like) may occur afterwards. Mild oral analgesia usually suffices but if this does not work it is essential to review possible causes, such as bowel perforation (also see below).

Phase Three – Embryology laboratory procedures

Phase Three commences in controlled laboratory conditions when a suitable egg and sperm have been retrieved.

Oocyte incubation

The eggs are initially incubated in a sterile culture medium, usually for some four hours, at a temperature of 37°C and in an atmosphere of 5 or sometimes 6% CO_2 (carbon dioxide).

Insemination

In IVF, 50,000-100,000 mature motile (moving purposefully) sperm are selected after being washed and added to mature-looking (metaphase 2 in development) oocytes. Usually each oocyte is treated separately. The mix is then returned to the controlled incubator environment.

In ICSI, single sperms are injected into single eggs from which the outer surrounding layer of cells (cumulus coronal complex) has been stripped away (see Figure 15, page 210).

Fertilisation

It is hoped fertilisation will begin in the next 12-15 hours (see chapter 2). Some 18 hours after insemination, visible changes can be seen under the microscope examination, with pronuclear development, and a preliminary verdict can usually then be given as to what is happening. But even if it looks good, there is no final guarantee that there will be anything suitable to transfer, as growth by cell division may stop or become abnormal.

Pre-implantation cell division and possible process interventions

Progress should continue to be reviewed microscopically. The number of cells in the embryo being transferred will depend on the days between insemination and transfer.

Assisted hatching

Assisted hatching is the technique where a hole is cut/lasered in the zona-pellucida (the skin of cells that surrounds the embryo). This can be done before the embryo is transferred to the uterus if implantation difficulties are anticipated, for example if the embryo shell is thick or when pregnancy has not occurred after repeated transfer of quality embryos. Whether it really influences matters is conjectural, except perhaps in older women with previously failed cycles but good quality embryos transferred.

Pre-implantation diagnosis(PGD) and screening(PGS).

Day 3 is the embryo age when blastomeres (1-2) can be removed for pre-implantation genetic diagnosis (PGD) if this is required and indicated by age, family or sibling history. Appropriate reliable laboratory facilities need to be available. Pre-preparation; involving counselling, advice from a clinical geneticist, and, where necessary, genetic analysis of the couple's blood; is all part of essential good practice.

Pre-implantation diagnosis started clinically in 1990 and is continuing to expand along with the science of genetics. Not all diseases with a genetic origin can yet be screened for. There may be a medical indication to examine the embryonal cells that have been removed for their sex and thus aid embryonal diagnosis of sex-linked disorders such as haemophilia and Duchenne muscular dystrophy. Chromosomal abnormalities may also be detected, such as in Down syndrome, and single gene disorders such as cystic fibrosis (CF). It can also make possible the creation of a 'saviour sibling'.

No technique in medicine is 100% effective and PGD is no exception. However, for those who may need it, although pregnancy rates are lowered, PGD can allow pre-transfer differentiation between those carrying a defect and those who are not, thus helping to prevent the birth of affected children. Follow-up with conventional prenatal diagnosis is still recommended.

Pre-implantation screening (PGS) using the same techniques as PGD has also been in vogue for some time. The reasons behind it are to try to improve pregnancy rates in those undergoing IVF by screening for possible abnormalities, though there is no specific genetic history to suggest there might be an increased chance of an offspring having a genetic abnormality. This is a somewhat different goal from PGD, where a specific history exists to justify the potential morbidity (damage) to the embryos and the consequences of decision-making on the basis of possible false positive or negative results that can sometimes occur where such invasive techniques are used. Some 60% of genetic abnormalities found are due to 'mosaicism' (the embryo has cells with different chromosome make-ups). Additionally, up to 50% of cleavage stage embryos with an aneuploidy (abnormality) that survive to the blastocyst stage, 'self correct'. The present consensus is therefore that employing such screening techniques for PGS as opposed to PGD is unjustified even though polar body biopsy (see chapter 2, page 4) and validated 24-hour chromosome analysis could be a way of overcoming such snags (ESHRE, 2009).

It is conjectural whether the future in these areas lies with pre-implantation genetic analysis of day 4 cells taken from the extra embryonic 'trophectoderm' part of the blastocyst (one of the two parts of the embryo that it has divided into by day 4 and which forms the embryonic part of the placenta as opposed to the other part, the inner cell mass, which will go on to form the post-implantation embryo: see chapter 2). This is currently under research examination but, at present, the time needed for proper genetic analysis of the cells requires the embryo to be frozen, with transfer on a subsequent cycle when the results have become available. This is somewhat impractical in the ordinary clinical setting.

Phase Four – Embryo transfer

Day 2 after egg collection (4-6 cell stage), or day 3 (6-10 cells), is the time most commonly used for embryo transfer, but blastocyst transfer (day 4-6) with multiple cells may be used in certain circumstances. Indeed, nowadays, in some clinics this can be the norm for the majority of cycles even though it involves more complex laboratory procedures and overall results are no better. Other units are more selective, preferring day 2-3 for transfer in most normal circumstances.

Medical indications where pregnancy rates may be improved by a blastocyst transfer include: an abnormally shaped uterus; a known weakness in the cervix; a history of twins on a previous IVF attempt; and where two earlier cycles have failed despite transfer of good quality embryos. Additionally, the HARI unit amongst others obtained eSET (single embryo transfer) figures of 50% in IVF 'good prognosis' patients.

Transfers, whatever the day, are performed without anaesthetic via the cervix using a thin tube (catheter) into which the embryo(s) selected for transfer have been loaded (see Figure 18, page 228).

The basic evaluation that all embryos normally undergo before being chosen for transfer at present relies on morphological (visual) appearance and cleavage (cell division) patterns. It is certainly imperfect. Although the highest grade embryos undoubtedly do best, all working in this area recognise that sometimes those graded highest may still fail unexpectedly whereas a much lower grade one manages to succeed. So for you to be totally hung up on the results of this 'beauty contest' can be unwise.

If the eventual aim is elective single embryo transfer (eSET), better criteria are needed. Perhaps the future in this regard may lie in combining present visual evaluations using better technology, such as polarised light microscopy, with totally non-invasive techniques that examine substances in the culture medium in which the embryo has been growing. These latter could be reflections of the embryo's metabolism and thus might help better assess its reproductive potential. A number of substances or processes have been examined, including pyruvate, glucose and amino acids.

Perhaps of greatest promise, but still totally experimental as with these other techniques and not yet available clinically, is the study (metabolomics), detection, and measurement of metabolites called metabolomes, which are a number of small molecules that have been observed to be biologically associated with specific physical or biochemical changes in the embryo (its functional 'phenotype') and are most likely determined by its genetic make-up.

At a technical level, the cervix is first visualised, as in IUI, using a vaginal speculum. The embryo(s) are transferred (released gently with the aid of a syringe) into the uterus between mid-part and to up to 1 cm from the fundus (bottom of the uterus). It is important that the person doing the transfer has been fully trained. Some find ultrasound helps position the catheter within the uterus.

Although not legislated for in all jurisdictions, the trend, especially in Europe, is to transfer a maximum of two embryos, with three in very exceptional circumstances. This may soon change; the aim now is to achieve a singleton baby from a single embryo transfer as the gold standard (see page 240). The number of embryos being transferred should be agreed between the clinic and the couple when the couple consent to treatment and this should be confirmed just before transfer when the number and quality of embryos available is known.

After a short rest (in some units none, in others 30 minutes) the woman can go home to normal life apart from taking luteal phase support – either hGG injections or more commonly daily proges-terone administrated vaginally as a gel or pessaries, or as injections prescribed for the next 14 to 16 days (see phase 5, page 233).

Potential complications in phases three and four of a treatment cycle

Nothing to transfer

Rarely, no eggs are found in the aspirated follicles (empty follicle syn-drome). Failure of some of the eggs harvested to be fertilised is common and has been reported in up to 50% of eggs obtained, depending on the woman's age. Failure of some embryos to keep growing sufficiently to be suitable for transfer is also relatively common; this has been reported in up to 25% of individual embryos, again depending on the woman's age. Even where embryos do get transferred, USA data show that eight out of ten fail to implant. Studies in my own clinic and elsewhere have shown that only some 3.6% of eggs harvested end up as a birth.

An egg's potential to be fertilised reduces by 50% over the age of 40. However, it is quite rare to have nothing to transfer in the fresh cycle that has just been undertaken, or to freeze if transfer needs to be delayed because no eggs were obtained or normal fertilisation failed completely. Nonetheless, leaving the time to transfer to the blastocyst developmen-tal stage increases the risk, as does undertaking PGD by removing one or more blastomere (embryonic cell) for genetic analysis.

The formation of a viable embryo is also dependent on sperm presence and quality including DNA integrity (pages 4, 215). Failure to produce a semen sample on demand for an IVF cycle may not always be antici-pated; if it is, it is essential to have a pre-frozen reserve sample available as a back-up. In azoospermia due to mechanical obstruction there is an

Figure 18 Diagrams of transfer

Diagram of female vagina/uterus'

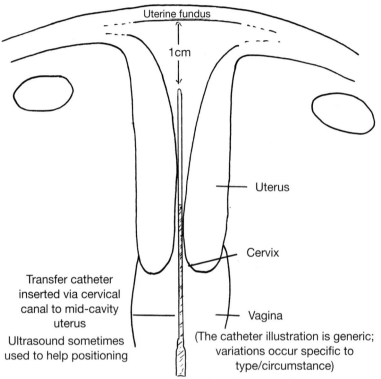

Uterine fundus

1cm

Uterus

Cervix

Transfer catheter inserted via cervical canal to mid-cavity uterus

Vagina

Ultrasound sometimes used to help positioning

(The catheter illustration is generic; variations occur specific to type/circumstance)

Lateral cross-section of pelvis at transfer

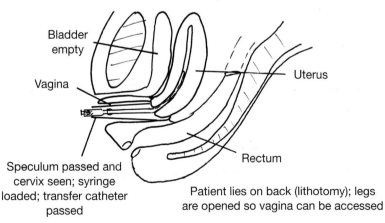

Bladder empty

Vagina

Uterus

Rectum

Speculum passed and cervix seen; syringe loaded; transfer catheter passed

Patient lies on back (lithotomy); legs are opened so vagina can be accessed

almost 100% chance of obtaining suitable sperm operatively (see pages 53, 212) compared with a chance of only 50% in azoospermia caused by other factors. But quality obtained may disimprove as age increases. In such situations it is necessary to be sure sperm will be available when required before embarking on a cycle of therapy; cryo-preservation of an earlier sample as insurance is advisable.

Complications at transfer

Transfer complications are rare, but the pregnancy rate is higher the less complicated the procedure has been, provided that the operatives performing it are equally adept. Transfer may need to be delayed if technical difficulties arise or the woman experiences pain. Torsion (twisting) of the ovary is very rare but also very painful. Analgesics are given and the embryos cryopreserved to enable transfer to be postponed.

Egg collection itself and the immediate aftermath can also be painful but rarely is the patient not up to transfer at that time leading to the need to freeze the embryos there and then (a 'freeze-all') with transfer at a later date when the patient feels better.

Embryo cryopreservation and storage

General

The first successful birth from a frozen and thawed embryo was in 1983. Results have improved with developments in cryopreservation. Storage of embryos until a future transfer date should now be provided for couples who wish and for whom the indications are appropriate. Thought is needed and discussion of the implications before enrolling in a cryopreservation/embryo storage programme. In particular, questions relating to potential future usage and length of storage need to be addressed. In most countries, it is thought wise to require both of the couple's informed consent to be given both initially pre-freeze and again pre-thaw and pre-transfer or disposal.

When to do it?

It would now be considered dangerous for an IVF clinic not to have an embryo freezing programme available to cope with instances where a 'freeze-all' is indicated on safety grounds, such as where ovarian hyperstimulation syndrome – OHSS – is very likely. If there are additional embryos available surplus to requirement for immediate transfer, these can be stored for future cycle usage, sparing the couple the full procedure should the present one not succeed or they wish to try to procreate again if it does.

Importantly, freezing allows the number of embryos transferred in one cycle to be reduced and with that, the chances of multiple pregnancy. In some countries, but not all, it also enables couples to donate stored embryos that have become irrevocably surplus to requirement to other couples (3%) or for research (59%) (2009 data). This is, however, totally dependent on the legislative regime of the country concerned.

Embryo freezing is arguably best attempted in the earlier stages of cell division (day 2-3) as soon as some idea of viable progress is identifiable. The extremes are: the two-pronuclear stage (day 1) and the blastocyst stage (day 4-6) at the latest, although growing on to this stage is more difficult and requires sequential changes of culture media.

Some countries (Germany and Switzerland), however, only allow cryopreservation at the very early, two pronuclear single-cell stage (20-22 hours after insemination: see also chapter 2) rather than after the embryo has started to divide. These freeze well but their quality has not been properly tested by observing cell division before they are frozen; unnecessary material giving false future hope may therefore be stored and the chances of a future pregnancy lessened .

Oocyte freezing

Now found unconstitutional in parts (2009) Italian law on IVF (2004) allowed only eggs to be frozen. This is more problematic as eggs are more susceptible to injury from freezing than embryos due to a higher water content. Two techniques are currently in use. The original method, called the slow freeze technique, is reasonably similar to that for freezing embryos, although different cryoprotectants are used. Results are improving from the original 1% to 2% in 2007 of live births per oocyte thawed, but egg attrition is still high. One unit in Italy in 2005 claimed a 13.9% pregnancy rate, but an average of 39 eggs seems to have been expended for each pregnancy achieved compared with 9.5 for frozen embryo success.

The other technique first used in humans in 1999 called vitrification is now coming into greater use for embryos, including blastocysts and eggs, although some questions as to ultimate safety still need final verification as high, possibly toxic, levels of cryoprotectant are used. It is said to be cheaper and because a flash freeze technique is used it is certainly quicker. Results are similar to those for frozen embryos. For eggs, the live birth rate /oocyte rapid thaw vitrification method has been reported in 2007 to be double that of the slow method at 4%.

Egg, or indeed ovarian tissue, freezing can also be used in women, as in men (see semen cryo-banking, chapter 7) to preserve their ability to have children in the future should the woman face a disease, especially cancer, where the disease or its treatment may destroy reproductive function.

The basic principles behind the freezing/storage/transfer process

Except with the vitrification method, the basic principle of freezing gametes and embryos is first to remove the water from the cells and replace it with a cryoprotectant to prevent ice-crystal formation and then gradually lower the temperature using liquid nitrogen until a temperature of -196°C is reached. The embryos are then stored in containers at this temperature in coded, identifiable (secure system) straws, one per receptacle, until required. Before thaw and transfer further signed and witnessed consent is needed by both man and woman. Embryos from couples who have tested positive for a virus should be stored separately, in quarantine.

Thawing the agreed number of embryos for transfer is simple. (Rules differ but a maximum of two, especially if the woman is under 40 years, is the norm for many centres worldwide.) This can be done the day before, allowing the viability of the embryos to be checked, or on the day of transfer itself.

After cross-checking the identity of the embryo, it is removed from its liquid nitrogen storage container and kept at room temperature for five minutes. This will suffice for thawing to be complete and to allow assessment of viability by the embryologist.

Transfer is as for a fresh cycle, timed at two to three days after ovulation if a natural cycle is being used. A pre-transfer check that the endometrial lining is sufficiently developed (9 mm thickness or more at ultrasound) is advisable. In some women adequate endometrial growth does not occur and for others, detecting ovulation time is difficult. Instead of a natural cycle a hormone-controlled cycle is an alternative.

Oestrogen can be given orally to promote endometrial development, initially for 10-12 days. If the endometrium does not grow sufficiently thick by then, the dosage can be increased or if the lining is under 7 mm thick the transfer can be postponed to a later date, with an adjusted dosage of oestrogen. In such cycles, for luteal support, progesterone is added to the oestrogen for 16 days. A pregnancy test is then done. This is because even if the woman is not pregnant,vaginal bleeding is unlikely to occur owing to the drugs until sometime later (withdrawal bleed). If the test is negative the drugs are then stopped but are continued on for a further 28 days if pregnancy has occurred.

Frozen cycle potential complications

Survival

Not all embryos survive freezing, storage and thawing. When freezing is on day 2-3, up to 78% may survive, fewer when on day 4-5. Sometimes, however, after thawing none survives, as can be seen if post-thaw viability and quality are checked the day before transfer, as in my own unit to avoid aimless waste of time. Because of this, in my clinic 30% of women in 2004 had nothing to transfer in their freezing cycle. The poorer the initial quality, and the fewer embryos available, the more likely this is to happen.

When freezing is performed at the pronuclear stage, transfer rates are shown to be lower at 68% compared with 79% for day 2-3 embryos. Where eggs are frozen, attrition rates are, as discussed above, even higher.

Wrong identification/transfer and freezer failure
Mis-identification has been reported despite assiduous controls being in place, as has freezer failure.

Viral transfer between straws
There is also the possibility of contamination between straws by viruses, although this has never been reported. It is for this reason that the clinic needs to determine the viral status of the couple some 30 days before starting, re-test afterwards (after 180 days) and quarantine all straws for those 180 days, prior to transfer to the main storage facility. Known viral positives should be kept separately grouped as per the virus throughout their frozen lives.

Phase Five – the 3-4 weeks after transfer

Down-regulation will affect the woman's own progesterone production, which sustains the early pregnancy. She will therefore need to take hormone supplements; the alternatives are daily progestogens given vaginally as a gel or pessary or by injection for 14-16 days, or hCG injections. Similar luteal support is given after frozen cycle transfers.

Access to the clinic for advice and to deal with any complications, if possible in-house, should be available during and after the cycle has been completed. Even if apparent failure is the result and vaginal bleeding starts, a urinary pregnancy test is wise. Although likely negative, there is always the possibility of a very early threatened miscarriage or an ectopic (especially tubal) pregnancy. Where the test result is negative, a post procedure review of everything should be carried out and decisions made as to what to do next.

If the test is positive, it is usual to suggest that early contact is made by the couple with their antenatal clinic of choice, to which full details should be sent by the IVF unit. Many clinics and couples like to have an early scan at around three weeks after a positive test so as to be reassured that the pregnancy is viable and to check how many embryos have successfully implanted. This is often easiest to arrange in the IVF clinic, whose staff should always be happy to see and record positive outcomes.

Potential complications after the cycle

Side effects complicating treatment are a significant factor in all infertility therapy however healthy the couple is usually; these can be particularly dangerous in IVF.

Ovarian hyperstimulation syndrome (OHSS)

The IVF/ICSI therapies call for very powerful stimulation of the ovaries in a deliberate attempt to obtain a number of mature follicles and from them mature eggs. This will inevitably lead to a small percentage of women experiencing ovarian hyperstimulation syndrome (OHSS, see also page 125). World published data show a variation in overall OHSS incidence from 0.6% to 14% (ESHRE 2004, 1.2%; HARI 1.9%).

The signs appear after egg collection, but sometimes the possibility may be raised before this if monitoring shows a large number of follicles developing during ovulation stimulation or levels of oestradiol quickly become very high. Symptoms may be mild with some abdominal swelling and pain. They may be moderate, with increased pain and swelling, through to severe. The severe form can even result in death in a number of ways. There can be acute painful ovarian enlargement and formation of ovarian cysts that may rupture or haemorrhage. Diarrhoea and vomiting can cause dehydration. There can be changes in coagulation factors, which can lead to excessive clotting, resulting in a blood clot (thromboembolism). Excess fluid can be formed in the abdomen (ascites) and sometimes in the chest (hydrothorax), which may be associated with respiratory failure (Adult Respiratory Distress Syndrome; ARDS).

The condition is self-limiting. Women with the mild form usually recover at home in a few days. Under 2% overall may need admission for fluid replacement and analgesia. Few of these, perhaps some 0.6% of the total, will develop the severe form requiring appropriate emergency measures.

Pregnancy may make the situation worse so, if OHSS is thought a very likely possibility and a decision has been made to give hCG or the alternatives rLH or GnRHa (see page 219) before proceeding to egg recovery, there should be no fresh transfer and a freeze-all is appropriate.

Failure

Failure is likely to be the norm for many couples (CDC USA, 2004: 66% of cycles do not produce a pregnancy). The clinic must give time for examining possible causes and then for full consultation with the couple as to why and what to do next. Sometimes the prognosis is clearly hopeless and couples need to be told this, however painful it may be. Counselling-out and other options need to be discussed. Sometimes it can be seen that a modification to the therapy based on the previous response can be considered. However, after undergoing three good cycle attempts with no success and no further therapy changes genuinely being appropriate, discontinuation and expert counselling-out may well be in the couple's best interests (see also chapter 13, pages 252-4).

Complications of pregnancies achieved

A number of the complications that can be found after natural conception may also occur post IVF. The incidence may be increased (see also chapter 13, pages 254-6). Up to 50%+ Caesarian section is common.

Miscarriage
Rates above the apparent norm (15-20%) have been reported by some following fresh IVF, but not by others (CDC 2004, 15.5%), and more so after frozen cycles (30%).

Ectopic pregnancy
Ectopic pregnancy may occur in up to 2% (HARI Clinic 2004, CDC 0.7%) even in the absence of tubes, as embryos are transferred from below and can stray into a tube stump from the uterus. This rate is higher than for spontaneous conceptions (Rotunda Hospital, Dublin 2004, 1%).

Perinatal mortality, morbidity and caesarean section
Increases have also been reported in perinatal mortality, injury and caesarean section. However, no pregnancy, however achieved, can be guaranteed complication-free. When corrected for age and the presence of multiple pregnancies, there does not appear to be a significant increase in perinatal mortality risk, in general terms, although singleton premature delivery is still twice normal for IVF pregnancies.

Abnormalities in offspring
Longer-term health studies of the offspring of IVF are limited but seem to suggest an increase in congenital malformations at birth with IVF/ICSI of the order of 1.3 to 1. The CDC reported certain birth defects to be two to four times more likely from IVF conceptions than from natural conceptions, especially cleft lip (2.4 times) and alimentary tract atresia (closure) (3.7-4.5 times) (Press Release, November 2008).

Age does increase the risk of chromosome defects. Not all of these are incompatible with life, as is the case with Down syndrome. The incidence of this in a woman at age 30 is around 1/909, at 40 1/112 and at 45 1/28. ICSI is thought possibly to contribute more than IVF to certain types of rare congenital abnormalities classified as 'imprinting defects'. This is by no means proven and the incidence is very low (0.1%). Blastocyst transfer does not seem to have reduced the incidence of pre-transfer chromosomal abnormality (aneuploidy) as significantly as had been hoped, but the implication of this in terms of normality at birth and thereafter is not always clear. Aneuploidy has been reported as being as high as 62% for fresh blastocysts and 75% when thawed from frozen.

Multiple pregnancy

A major risk to mother and child after IVF is multiple pregnancy (ESHRE 2003, 26%; CDC 2004, 33.5%) and delivery (ESHRE 2004, 22.7%; CDC, 26.7% of fresh non-donor deliveries) particularly those of a high order (3+: ESHRE 2004, 1%; CDC, 2.6%). Desperate couples will welcome any pregnancy. Twins (30% of all twin births are from IVF) are often seen as the ideal solution. However, mostly due to the associated increase in premature birth, the presence of a multiple pregnancy compounds every complication throughout pregnancy for mother and fetus, and after birth, the neonatal period and beyond (see also chapter 13).

It really is the quality of embryos available for transfer that matters. Age is important. Egg and embryo quality drop in women over 40. Up to 40 years, expected pregnancy rates from IVF can be maintained by transferring a maximum of two embryos and at 30 years, by transferring electively (eSET) only one quality embryo, although others have reported up to 9% lower rates.

Transfer policies to avoid multiple pregnancies are now under scrutiny worldwide. While 'fetal reduction' is still offered by some, for many it is not an alternative to be considered. Fetal reduction is the euphemism used to describe a technique that some units in some countries offer when multiple embryonal sacs are seen to have implanted. A drug that is lethal to the embryo is injected under ultrasound control into some of the sacs, thus terminating the life within them. This achieves the aim of reducing the number of ongoing pregnancies. It is not without hazard and for many is tantamount to abortion and unacceptable.

Stress
Some couples find the whole ART programme particularly trying. There are specific stress points along the journey from initial acceptance, but in the end, prognosis does not appear to be affected by stress as far as IVF conception is concerned. Appropriate clinical ambience, information and education, plus the clinic being on the look-out for signs of excessive stress and providing appropriate counselling, seem to help (see chapter 10, pages 168-70).

Prognosis for success – results

General

Interpreting what the true pregnancy and take-home baby rates are for a specific clinic can be very problematic for a couple. Age is the most important prognostic factor and overall figures can be biased by a preponderance of young women at a particular clinic. Good clinics show success rates for the different average female age bands.

A similar situation occurs where clinics have careful selection policies and cherry-pick couples who are likely to be easy to treat; their figures will be very different from those clinics, such as the author's, that take all comers for whom IVF is indicated and who are suitable. A busy clinic with well-trained, experienced personnel usually does best. The number of cycles performed per annum may help a potential couple judge this.

Pregnancy should always be verified by ultrasound, not just by the initial urine test. Early but transient raised urinary hCG levels may give false positive results (the 'biochemical pregnancy').

Spontaneous conceptions, 'the background placebo effect', can occur. Rates of some 11% overall have been reported, and 16% if men with azoopermia and women with tubal-factor infertility – that is, those who really can never conceive naturally – are excluded. Similarly, I and others have found that 21% of couples who have an IVF success (excluding those with azoospermia and tubal-factor infertility) get pregnant again naturally within two years. These 'placebo-type' spontaneous pregnancies should not be included in clinic success figures.

Statistics

All statistics are potentially open to differences in interpretation and to manipulation. In what in most of the world is a competitive and potentially exploitative private practice market, clinics perhaps understandably try to present their results as positively as possible. Couples need to read the figures supplied carefully. How the results are stated is important, particularly the age profile, and the end point used and whether comparisons are like-for-like and verifiable.

Pregnancy rates can be calculated in a number of ways – per single cycles of treatment or over a period of time or number of cycles (cumulative). Because of the attrition occurring during the cycle, rates per

IVF cycle started will be lower than per egg retrieval procedure and lower again than per transfer (cycle completed or ET). Pregnancy rates will be higher than take-home baby rates (the live birth of at least one baby weighing at least 500 grams) for the same reason.

Examples of potential manipulation can occur, especially with blastocyst results. Rates are invariably quoted per transfer (ET) rather than per cycle started or per egg collection. If these other parameters were used instead, the 50%+ often quoted would be lower and, indeed, due to increased risk of no-transfer, prognosis could well be lower in most circumstances than using a day 2-3 transfer instead. Not counting cancelled cycles, adding in multiple pregnancies as more than one success (this is not truly the live birth rate), not separating out cycles where donor gametes were used, and adding in a subsequent frozen success so that it appears to come from the initial fresh stem cycle, are further manipulations sometimes practised to make a clinic look good.

However, at the end of the line, when looking at results in order to make a decision as to 'what next', bear in mind the USA's CDC very wise 2004 rider: 'a comparison of clinic success rates may not be meaningful because patient medical characteristics and treatment approaches vary from clinic to clinic.'

Fresh IVF/ICSI

The overall figures are thought to have improved somewhat over the years, little by little. The CDC in the USA (2005) quoted live birth rates per fresh non-donor transfers in 1996 of 28%, compared with 34% in 2005. However, there may now be a tailing off as this was almost the same rate as reported in 2003 and 2004 as well. ESHRE 2004 also shows an increase in pregnancy rates of almost 1% between 2003 and 2004, but actually a slight decrease in live birth rates from 21.7% to 20.6%. Such annual fluctuations may appear even greater in single clinic figures where from any single year to the next changes in the population served, the clinic personnel and practice may influence end results. This annual fluctuation is illustrated by the respective combined IVF/ICSI pregnancy and live birth per transfer figures for the HARI clinic at the Rotunda Hospital Dublin (Annual Reports, 2004: 35.2% and 29.4%; 2005, 36% and 31.9%; 2006, 33% and 28.7%; and 2007, 48.4% and 39.6%). Not all can be accounted for by practice changes of the European Tissue and Cell Directive 2004. The mean age of the women actually rose from 35.5 in 2004 to 36.1 in 2007. I have been 'assured' by the rest of an almost unchanged staff that my retirement had 'absolutely' nothing to do with the changes seen! In any clinic, steady improvement (speed does not matter, consolidation does) in verifiable annual unit returns, presented in a clear understandable manner is the reassurance that the discerning couple need to enquire about and be able to see.

Internationally, however, natural cycle IVF has stayed at around 7% per cycle. Modified natural IVF and mild IVF get somewhat higher results (in the teens), but as yet not as high as conventional IVF, though potentially less problematic. Those couples who have had a previous successful pregnancy seem to do better.

Where the gold-standard concept of a single baby from a single transferred embryo via elective single embryo transfer (eSET) has been applied in high numbers, such as in Finland, Denmark, Sweden and Belgium, live birth rates per transfer have not been worse than elsewhere. The woman's age and selection of the best embryo from those available for transfer seem to be the key.

For conventional IVF/ICSI, individual local clinics often seem to publish better figures than those quoted overall nationally or internationally. Smaller numbers may inflate percentages. International statistics give baseline pregnancy and delivery rates, but may not be up to date and also consolidate into one figure the best and the worst clinics. The overall volume tends to iron out gross fluctuations. They are, however, the best reflection of what can genuinely be achieved and of trends of change.

The most recently published ESHRE annual report, for 2004 (the seventh since 1997, found in *Human Reproduction* 2008; 123(4): 756-771 2008) does just this. The data supplied and tabulated from the reporting countries allow pan-European results from 281,864 fresh and 71,997 frozen cycles to be calculated for various ART activities in individual countries. The CDC report does the same for the USA (available from 1996-2006). In 2004 (see http://apps.nccd.cdc.gov/ART2004) 94,242 fresh and 18,560 cycles were started.

Both these reports are in some instances incomplete; some sections contain data from small numbers of various ART procedures that the compilers have put together under a single general heading for convenience. Some of the ESHRE/HARI figures have had to be extrapolated. You the reader need to understand all this when perusing tables that give IVF and ICSI success rates consolidated into one, as per the USA methodology.

My intention in quoting all this information is solely to give you as accurate an overall picture as is possible given the constraints on information available. Purely to illustrate in greater depth than previously shown on page 240 how any clinic can fluctuate considerably, I have included published HARI clinic data for both 2004 and 2007. Even though further reference to the source documents will provide more information, you cannot make any valid comparisons or draw conclusions from this or any other single clinic figures with data shown in the tables for ESHRE and CDC where the results depicted are, as stated on page 239, simply consolidations of both good and bad to achieve a mean or average. In order to conform with the like-for-like rule, wherever possible, the extrapolated figures in the following tables (1-3) relate to fresh non-donor cycles, IVF and ICSI together.

For international comparative purposes, 2004 has been selected, as at the time of going to print this was the last available year for all sources, but as stated previously, if you wish to know what the situation is today, in terms of large multi-sourced results, there has been very little change in prognosis if any since 2004.

It is clear that the results shown in Table 1 from the CDC/USA are better for achieving pregnancy than the overall results from Europe. Many attempts have been made to show why, the differences in practice and the differing contexts of this practice being two contributory factors. Multiple pregnancy rates post IVF are considerably higher in the USA (33.6 CDC, 2004), reflecting a different transfer policy to Europe

Table 1 Percentage of pregnancies and live births from fresh non-donor eggs IVF/ICSI cycles, egg collections and embryo transfers.

Source	Pregnancies			Live births		
	Per cycle	Per collection	Per transfer	Per cycle	Per collection	Per transfer
ESHRE 2004 281864 cycles	26.7	26.9	31	17.8	19.1	26.6
CDC 2004 94742 cycles	33.7	38.5	41.5	27.7	31.6	34
HARI 2004 856 cycles	28.7	32.7	34.9	23.7	27.0	29.4
HARI 2007 893 cycles	37.2	43.4	48.5	30.4	35.4	39.6

(ESHRE 26% in 2004, with HARI 25%). The USA CDC data are produced under a single set of national guidelines whereas the international data from ESHRE have to contend with many different sets of rules, some of which stand in the way of best practice and drag down the overall averages for other countries/clinics whose results bear good comparison with those from the USA.

Perhaps to attempt to make inter-country comparisons at all is non-productive for everyone but those who would wish to indulge in reproductive tourism.

Age plays a very important part in prognosis. The 2004 CDC (Table 2) and HARI (Table 3) data show this clearly even though the cut-off age points chosen are different. The tables show results per cycle started and per ET. The ESHRE data do not allow any such detailed analyses

Table 2 Percentage of pregnancies, live births fresh non-donor eggs IVF/ICSI, age divided per cycle and embryo transfer (CDC 2004)

	Pregnancies				
Age	<35	35-37	38-40	41-42	42+
Per cycle	42.5	35.5	26.5	17.3	8
Per embryo transfer	N/A	N/A	N/A	N/A	N/A
	Live births				
Per cycle	36.9	29.3	19.5	10.7	4
Per embryo transfer	42.7	35.5	25.3	14.8	8

Table 3 Percentage of pregnancies, live births fresh non-donor IVF/ICSI, age divided per cycle and embryo transfer (HARI 2004/2007)

	Pregnancies							
Age	<30		30-34		35-39		40+	
Year	2004	2007	2004	2007	2004	2007	2004	2007
Per cycle	41.4	31.1	33.6	47.0	26.7	38.7	17.5	22.7
Per embryo transfer	44.5	45.1	39.4	55.0	34.2	51.1	24.4	32.0
	Live births							
Per cycle	36.3	26.6	28.1	42.6	20.5	32.9	12.4	9.6
Per embryo transfer	39.1	38.7	32.9	50.0	26.3	43.5	17.3	13.6

to be tabulated. Transfer numbers drop with age. Far fewer get that far (CDC <35 years 86%, 42+ years 64%). This, however, will decrease the percentage chances of success in the over 40 age group.

Frozen embryo transfer success rates

It is not possible from reports to differentiate between stages of development when embryos were frozen. Additionally, some clinics transfer

Table 4 Percentage of pregnancies and live births per cycle and embryo transfer – non-donor frozen cycles

Source	Pregnancies		Live births	
	Per cycle	Per embryo transfer	Per cycle	Per embryo transfer
ESHRE 2004 71997 cycles	18.5	19.1	12.3	14.1
CDC 2004 18560 cycles	N/A	N/A	27.0	27.7
HARI 2004 326 cycles	19.3	27.9	14.1	20.4
HARI 2007 350 cycles	24.9	29.4	18.3	21.6

immediately post thaw, others check viability first. However, it is clear that frozen embryo cycle and transfer success rates are lower than fresh. Quality of the pre-freeze embryo is very important.

Frozen egg usage success rates

As discussed above in the freezing oocyte section, at present usage success rates vary between 2% and 4% live birth per oocyte (egg) thawed. However, recent improvements with vitrification are claimed to be double the slow-freeze method, where rates of 14% are now claimed.

PGD cycles

In appropriately selected patients where PGD (pre-implantation genetic diagnosis) has been used for a valid medical indication and normal (euploid) embryos transferred, an accuracy rate of 97-98% was found in the follow-up data of the first ten years pioneering practice. Services offering this technique have expanded, enlarging the data set, as demand for screening (PGS) has increased. In PGS, however, as previously stated above, the risk does not appear justified (see page 224) and demand for this reason will fall and be replaced by non-invasive methods.

Although biopsy for PGD when an embryo is at the 8-cell stage may not detrimentally affect its further growth, only one in four such biopsied embryos is capable of implantation, and euploidy (normality) found then in one cell may not be representative nor aneuploidy (abnormality) persist from then on, or be significant to fetal normality thereafter. In the ESHRE figures for 2004, 2701 such cycles were started with 1849 transfers overall in some 12 countries, with 42.7% pregnancies and 17.9% deliveries per transfer.

Personal Comment

IVF has transformed the prognosis for many couples. It should be an available option for all suitable infertile couples regardless of affordability. Upwards of 1% of babies now being delivered throughout the world have been conceived through IVF. We have learned a great deal, but we may be reaching the limits of achievable success with present methodology. IVF is not a one-stop cure-all. Beware of those who consider and advocate it as such. It is not always suitable and in many instances should not be the first treatment to be considered.

It is not, I feel, in the interests of a couple's health to undergo multiple attempts (more than three) that repeatedly end in failure without questioning why and accepting counselling-out before considering one more go. IVF is best utilised at the end of the line and when specifically indicated; otherwise it can in unscrupulous hands become a very stressful, expensive means of exploiting desperate, vulnerable couples who will try anything.

For safety's sake, embryo cryopreservation must be available. Egg and ovarian tissue freezing may yet prove to be techniques that preserve reproductive capability in women as efficiently as in men. Modified natural cycles and milder stimulation protocols could well be the way forward in the future and even at present may be preferable in selected cases.

Pre-implantation diagnosis for genetic abnormality (PGD) is on the increase. Risk/benefit analysis comes out on the side of positive: PGD can be invaluable in preventing some serious genetic disorders from being passed on; but its use should be confined to the detection of serious disorders and a careful regulatory watch kept to prevent trivial or eugenically motivated abuse. Screening, on the other hand (PGS), using the same methods is now considered too risky but non-embryo-invasive methods are under development and cannot come too soon if embryos giving the best chance of successful pregnancy are to be identified for transfer.

Internationally collected results seem often to bear little resemblance to the publicity surrounding data that appear in the media or are put out by clinics themselves. Even in the USA at least two thirds of couples undergoing a cycle will not conceive. End-point parameters used by individual clinics are often picked to put them in the best possible light, so read any data provided to you carefully.

Multiple pregnancies, especially high order, can be a disastrous drain on all, but despite the adverse publicity even in respect of twins, the feeling of most infertile couples going into IVF after many years without children is that this is the optimum outcome and they can then pack up the quest. If appropriate experienced antenatal and neonatal care is available, a degree of emotional support can be provided in these circumstances, but given all the increased complications of twin pregnancies, this belief is not supportable medically.

Chapter 12

Alternative therapies

MYTHS

All alternative medicine is useless!
Any alternative medicine is the best approach!

Background

The media in all its guises abounds with descriptions of diets, complementary therapies and alternative medicines that are alleged to help the infertile conceive. The treatment that is promoted is seldom if ever backed up by proper scientific evidence. Results are rarely capable of being replicated and whether the successes claimed are greater than the placebo effect is not determined. Much more research is necessary to prove any of these approaches is effective beyond a positive placebo effect. Cost effectiveness is rarely if ever discussed or written about and the sums of money you are asked to spend can be very considerable compared with conventional practice.

What is available, its use and possible prognosis

Dietary supplements

While having a good diet is essential for general and reproductive health, from time to time reports surface promoting increased fertility rates associated with particular diets and foods, especially mineral and vitamin supplements. The list is long and varied. Many concern metals, such as zinc, to improve sperm counts, for example. There is little hard evidence on this subject, but the soy food isoflavone has been found to depress sperm counts.

It is claimed that vitamin E deprivation can cause sterility in humans but specific evidence is scanty in what is always a multi-factorial situation. Side effects exist. Too much vitamin A may cause erectile dysfunction and embryo damage; early fears about excessive vitamin C affecting cervical mucus have not, however, been substantiated.

Folic acid and vitamin B12 supplements have been scientifically shown to help prevent neural-tube defects such as spina bifida and, more recently, possibly miscarriage. All women intending to try for a pregnancy should be taking them.

Therapies with some basis in a relaxation effect

There are many therapies that promote relaxation, including yoga, transcendental meditation (TM) and autogenic training to name but three. Whichever is chosen by the individual, the latter two in particular have been shown in well-designed scientific studies to help relieve psychological and biochemical manifestations of stress in infertile couples (see page 171); however, some can find the trappings, costs, and mysticism surrounding in particular transcendental meditation not to be to their liking. Brain function may be altered (neuroplasticity) and achieving the so-called 'relaxation response' can help people be more content and stable in their daily lives. Pregnancies have been claimed to follow but true placebo-controlled studies in infertility do not exist.

There is no real potential to do harm, stress can be relieved and there is no reason why any of the many formats available cannot be used alongside conventional medicine.

Healing therapies

The healing therapies include aromatherapy, reflexology, iridology, crystal, stone and magnetic therapies plus bio-energy healing. Some of these may have a relaxation component that contributes to how it is claimed they work. Successes are quoted but, other than a placebo-type effect possibly associated with the ritual involved, the touching, and the time and support given, it is hard to see how these can work. This is not to say that they cannot work, but although anecdotally pregnancies do occur, none of the above methods has been found to have proven worth in the infertility situation when attempts have been made to test them scientifically.

It is worth noting that reflexology and some of the essences used in aromatherapy are not recommended by some practitioners for use in pregnancy.

Acupuncture

Acupuncture is popular, in widespread use and advocated for many conditions. It has arguably been the most researched of all complementary and alternative therapies and has many advocates and practitioners amongst 'main-stream' medical professionals. It has been used for many centuries in Chinese medicine to cure a wide range of ills and as an alternative to anaesthetic. Scientific study has found it can help back pain. Indeed, when the wrist pressure point (P6 Neguain, the No 6 Meridian point on the pericardial channel) is stimulated by a wrist bead, pelvic pain after IVF egg-collection has been shown to be relieved better than with a sham control.

Recent in-depth analysis of studies involving 1366 women compared acupuncture with controls (sham acupuncture or none) at embryo transfer and found a positive effect, with acupuncture increasing the odds of pregnancy by 65%. This has been interpreted as meaning that 10 women need to be treated with acupuncture to give one additional pregnancy. Overall, however, acupuncture seems optimally employed in situations best described as 'placebo responsive', a term which definitely includes infertility. The fact that the couple feel they are doing something may contribute to this helpful effect.

Visitations

There are many devotees of the positive power of prayer or of visiting a specific shrine for infertility, as for other medical conditions. There is no scientific evidence that this can help, but it can do little harm.

Plant and animal extracts

Yohimbine, extracted from an African tree bark, continues to be successful in treating male erectile dysfunction (see chapter 10, page 153). Anti-oxidants given in combination with linseed, vitamin B_6 and zinc have recently been suggested to improve sperm motility.

Other preparations, often Chinese in origin, carry with them powerful messages of increasing fertility potential that have built up since time immemorial. Placebo studies do not exist. The worry with all such medicines is being sure of their content and what the quality control mechanisms for their manufacture are. This uncertainty increases the potential for adverse interactions between traditional medicines, and between a traditional medicine and any of the conventional drugs being used. The traditional medicine could also have embryogenic and toxic effects on the early pregnancy. While certainly in successful use in their countries of origin, and indeed worldwide by complementary medicine practitioners, the uncertainty as to content, purity and manufacturing quality control makes the use of traditional medicines for infertility unwise, even as a placebo. Of interest, a recent as yet unpublished study from HARI found 46% of patients admitted regular use of herbal remedies, with 39% in the three months prior to IVF treatment.

Personal Comment

To strive to do no harm is the keystone of all medical practice but it is important to be aware people with vested interests may over-sell a specific alternative solution. However, if an alternative or complementary approach has been shown to have no ill-effects and may contribute to a positive result, either directly or via a placebo effect, it should not be ruled out. Research has shown that stress can be helped by some relaxation therapies and that these can be a valuable adjunct to conventional infertility treatment, whether a child is conceived or not.

Chapter 13

Coping with negative and positive outcomes

MYTHS

1. Not getting pregnant is in all ways a total disaster.
2. Achieving pregnancy is everything; after that it's plain sailing.

Potential positives about a negative result

Not all couples who embark on infertility investigations and treatment will end up having their own baby. Indeed, it was shown pre-IVF that the majority of couples seeking help (up to 70%) did not conceive. This has improved very little today. A small chance of conception, however, still continues for most people throughout their reproductive years, where conception is not completely blocked. It is therefore foolish to suggest there is never a chance.

Some problems have a better prognosis than others given time. In 'unexplained infertility', for instance, one recent study showed 22% of women had subsequently conceived out of the blue after four years of trying, and around 14% after two years of clinic attendance had been completed (see also chapter 10, pages 175-6). A spontaneous conception is not unknown after treatment has failed and been stopped (IVF 6%) or even a number of years later (1% up to 10 years). But there does come a time when continuing attendance and treatment may not benefit the situation over and above what can be achieved by prayer, or a visit to a shrine.

Basic management

Where no pregnancy has occurred despite the best efforts of all involved, the clinic should make special efforts to ensure the quality of the couple's life is not to be damaged. Time should be allowed and opportunities given for alternatives to be discussed. The first step is to suggest doing nothing more. It is not obligatory to have a child.

Some couples will find this an appropriate solution, especially if they were ambivalent about the whole issue at the outset and had bowed to external pressures in embarking on trying for a child. Helping both partners to counsel-out when a couple wish to discontinue is important. It helps them get back to their normal lives and breaks the vicious circle of going from clinic to clinic in search of their aim.

Getting round the problem

When a cause is diagnosed that totally rules out a conception from one or both of the partner's gametes, or the suggested treatment is unacceptable or has repeatedly failed and nothing more can be offered, this is not necessarily the end of the help that can be given.

Donor gametes and embryos

Donor gametes can be either sperm or eggs. The possibility of finding donor embryos should be discussed with the clinic.

Surrogacy

Surrogacy may be a solution for some, including male couples, where is it impossible (no uterus) or dangerous for the woman to carry a baby herself.

Adoption

Adoption has long been the answer for many childless couples.

Worldwide, there are still many abandoned babies and children whose lives could be transformed by this alternative. Numbers are highest in the developing world but often accessibility is made lengthy and bureaucratically difficult. Some feel taking a child outside its own culture is wrong.

Despite the difficulties, foreign adoption is the more likely route in most countries. In Ireland, for instance, which can be taken as typical of many countries' experiences, in 1991 there were 61 foreign adoptions; in 2003 there were 358, despite the increase in births outside marriage. Quoting again the Irish figures, in 1989 12.6% of babies were born to unmarried mothers compared with 31.4% in 2003. Both are an underestimate of potential as the number of women having pregnancy terminations outside the state needs to be factored in. However, the number of indigenous babies for adoption in this same country is miniscule compared with what it was before. In 1991 this was 590 (6.6%) and in 2003 only 92 (1.3%). Other countries where keeping the baby is also no longer a social stigma and is encouraged have similar figures.

Fostering

Fostering can for some be a realistic but of course temporary option to relieve the childlessness and can provide great help to children needing a secure home at difficult times in their lives. Levels have dropped in Ireland as in many other countries.

Problems that may occur with success

Achieving pregnancy does not guarantee a live baby. Unforeseen problems may spoil the party.

Medical complications

Miscarriage, ectopic pregnancy, fetal abnormality, and perinatal mortality may all be increased, especially if multiple pregnancy is involved.

All studies also report an increase in prematurity or caesarean section deliveries (over 50% of births after IVF). While all can go perfectly, couples must be briefed about these potential obstetric issues before fertility treatment and again before the baby's birth. This should be in all fertility situations, but especially after ovulation induction and IVF/ ICSI where multiple pregnancy (including high order, 3+) is commoner even despite nature itself reducing some 6% to a lesser number by one or more sacs not continuing on. Data show a significant increase in all complications of pregnancy, labour and afterwards to the mother, twins all grow slower. Birthweight is less than for infertility singletons, with half born before 37 weeks. Fifty percent are admitted to an ICU with chances of dying in the first week up to 6 times higher than for a singleton and 4 times the risk of cerebral palsy. Later they seem more frequently to have behavioural, language, visual and auditory impairments.

Unexpected further success

One success may be followed by another, spontaneously and quickly. For example, it has been shown that some 21% of couples with unexplained infertility who successfully conceive with IVF may have a second pregnancy spontaneously within two years. If this is not wanted or medically unwise, contraception should be part of the briefing process following successful delivery.

Parenting

Bringing up any child can have its problems. Multiple pregnancy can be rewarding but exhausting. Milestones reached late can be stressful and worrisome. This is more likely when the children are premature or have abnormalities, which can of course hold for singletons too.

Worry has been voiced about difficulties in parenting, arising especially in the older long-term infertile couple. Control studies suggest that these concerns are unfounded. However, advice and counselling on this subject may be important in helping couples to cope with this abrupt change in lifestyle and the fear that such a small and apparently delicate new arrival can engender in the new parents.

Personal Comment

Just when you think you can leave worries about infertility behind and can enjoy potential parenthood, a complication may come along and change that feeling. This possibility must not be forgotten; celebrations can be premature. It is the clinic's job to help and support couples in as safe a manner as possible, whether it is to maximise their experience of success and perhaps mention they may need contraception, or to advise and help with alternative approaches, or to counsel-out in the face of continued childlessness and with nothing more truly to offer whether the infertility has been alleviated or not. The clinic's role is to help couples make the most of the hand they have been dealt.

Chapter 14

Further sources of information

MYTH

What you read on the web or in a magazine is packed full of irrefutable facts. You hardly need a doctor at all.

Self-help groups

For those who do not mind disclosure of problems to others, joining a self-help group can help a lot. Usually, unbiased information will be available on many issues, and guidance given through written pamphlets and seminars. Meeting others in the same predicament can help when you are feeling you are the only ones who are infertile or have a specific problem.

Internet chat-rooms and pages are in some ways a modern solution to the self-help group where anonymity can be preserved, although sometimes groups and real supportive friendships can grow from this anonymous start. But, just as with any treatment, there is always a time to move on if obsession is not to become a problem.

Websites and other media sources

In addition to the information that can be gleaned from your family doctor and any clinics you attend, you may find the websites of the various clinics useful to see what is out there. Recent Irish Health Research Board Data have shown that overall some 1 in 4 patients seek website information. This is likely to be higher in present-day infertile couples as their age profile fits that of an aware, computer-literate generation.

Typing the word 'infertility' into a search engine can raise much information locally and internationally, but, like anything on the net, you need to be cautious about believing the claims made by those who wish to monitor apparent 'scientific advances'. The majority are on non-peer-reviewed sites where everyone is selling something.

Care needs to be taken in assessing the answers provided by interactive sites. The research findings quoted may not even be human data and what is said may not refer to or be suitable for your specific case. The same caveats go for other media information sources such as magazines, radio and TV programmes.

Internet reliables

'Internet reliables' are those websites that belong to national or international organisations involved in the area, with little or no bias. These include organisations such as:

IFFS (the International Federation of Fertility Societies – www.iffs-reproduction.org);

ESHRE (the European Society of Human Reproduction and Embryology – www.eshre.com);

ASRM (the American Society of Reproductive Medicine – www.asrm.org);

FIGO (the International Federation of Gynaecologists and Obstetricians – www.figo.org);

RCOG (the Royal College of Obstetricians and Gynaecologists – www.rcog.org.uk);

ISMAAR (the International Society for Mild Approaches in Assisted Reproduction – www.ismaar.org);

Centres for Disease Control and Prevention (ART data section) www.cdc.gov/art;

WHO (the World Health Organisation – www.who.int)
The Health on the Net Foundation - www.hon.ch

The main subscribable scientific journals specific to the general area of infertility include:
Fertility and Sterility (Elsevier) ASRM news.enquire via www.asrm.org;
Human Reproduction and its update.enquire via www.oxfordjournals.org.

Self-help groups include:
www.infertilityireland.ie;
www.fertilityfriends.co.uk;
www.resolve.org.

Other literature

Some clinics and government information bureaux provide information to couples. Perusal of a good bookshop will show many written alternatives exist. All will reflect some bias based on practice experience, as does this work, and the printed word in book form can soon go out of date.

Personal Comment

> *Clinics should be pro-active not only in providing their own informative web pages but also in guiding couples to reliable websites.*
>   *I find search engines such as google an excellent way of finding an easily understood definition for a specific technical*

word or phrase. I hope you will too. However, unlike a con-sultation, typing a single word such as 'infertility' to start an internet-search can provoke an indiscriminate response. You may find that chat-rooms can be full of unfounded negativity about specific clinics and participants often suggest therapies to each other. Supportive relationships can, however, develop between participants and group meetings can result. Unfil-tered information trawled by couples or on interactive sites may be misinterpreted as knowledge appropriate for them, when those with actual medical training will know it is not. For some of you this may cause anxiety (cyberchondria) and even sometimes unnecessary clashes with the clinic. 'Instant experts' are difficult to treat, especially when the information gained is of doubtful veracity. Infertility is, however, of great interest. The internet is here to stay.

Chapter 15

Epilogue – what does the future hold?

In this fast-moving specialty, who can properly predict what the future will hold even in the next few years? Will a more equitable method of funding infertility services for all those in need come into being? Maybe, as in the past, some new therapy as yet not even on the horizon will transform the prognosis for treating an abnormality in some part of the fertility profile, thus making 'there is more to infertility treatment than IVF' even more true? ART and especially IVF in all its guises is, however, likely to be a treatment option for a long time to come. In terms of IVF results, a plateau seems to have been reached. Moving on, if nature deems it possible, awaits a new initiative or discovery. Medically, the drive will be towards a single pregnancy from a single egg in IVF. Ovarian stimulation treatments will certainly continue but the need for a more selective approach will encourage the development of simpler, milder, improved and more cost-effective ovulation induction schemes overall. In IVF, a change in patients' attitude to multiple pregnancy and better identification and screening of oocyte and embryo quality is needed for elective single embryo transfer to become universal. Adding to morphological characteristics (appearance and growth patterns) by non-invasive techniques under the umbrella of 'metabolomics' and its like (the 'omics') may help this come to pass.

Oocyte freezing will improve and come into its own. Easier and more acceptable methods of prenatal diagnosis will become available, enabling more embryonic abnormalities to be detected. Whatever else happens, the old problems and longings for a baby, here since mankind began, will certainly continue as will our failure to be able to guarantee stress-free success at all times. There will still, for a few, be the occasional pleasant surprise 'out of the blue', when all active treatment and hope of a conception have long gone.

Index

Index

Index

Index

266

Index

counselling *(cont'd)*
  formal types
    behavioural therapy 156-8, 161-3
    psychodynamic 156, 161
  sensate focusing 157, 161
  indications for
    addiction 17
    AID 198
    genetic 52, 188
    IVF 171, 213, 237
    male, no therapy possible 53
    miscarriage, recurrent 192
    ovulation 131
    sexual dysfunction 151
    stress 171
    tubal surgery/IVF alternatives 86
  PCOs weight management 131
  psychotherapy, male 154-8
  psychotherapy, female 160-2
cryo-preservation
  see also in-vitro fertilisation
  complications, potential
    of eggs 230-1, 244
    of embryos 225, 243-4
    of semen 41, 57, 203, 208
  success rates 243-4
  transfer frozen cycle 232
cryptorchidism 40, 59
cycle monitoring *see* in-vitro fertilisation

D & C *see* dilation and curettage
definitions related to infertility (World Health Organisation (WHO))
  adenomyosis 104
  adhesions 64
  anti-sperm antibodies 50
  artificial insemination 194
  assisted reproduction techniques (ART) (WHO) 194
  fibroids 89
  infertility (WHO) 9
  internal endometriosis 104
  IVF (WHO) 209
  miscarriage, recurrent (WHO)182
  PCOs 129-30
  semen, abnormal 39
  semen, normal 49, 50

definitions related to infertility *(cont'd)*
  unexplained infertility (WHO) 32, 173
DES *see* diethylstilboestrol syndrome
diabetes
  fibroids, association with 90
  infertility, association with 48
  male 46, 48, 49
  miscarriage, recurrent 183, 187
  overweight 10, 187
  PCOs 129, 131, 133
diet 15, 22, 214, 247-8
dietary supplements 15, 55, 247-8
  see also alternative therapies
  anti-oxidants 59, 250
  folic acid 15, 22, 214, 248
  isoflavone 248
  linseed oil 250
  negative effect 43, 248
  positive benefit 247-8, 250
  vitamins 15, 180, 214, 248
  yohimbine 153, 250
  zinc 248
diethylstilboestrol syndrome (DES) 65
dilation and curettage (D & C) 71, 118
DIY
  AID 198-8
  AIH 203, 205
  alternative therapies 247-50
  de-stressing 169
  doing nothing 175
  home tests
    ovulation 23-4, 116-17
    male 23, 49
donor
  eggs 127, 213, 253
  embryos 230
  sperm 53, 196
dopamine agonists 126, 153
down regulation *see* IVF
drugs, street 17, 43, 51, 112, 150, 183
  see also cocaine, heroin, lifestyle, marijuana
  female, effect on 17, 159
  male, effect on 17,43,150
  miscarriage and 183
  ovulation and 112
  sexual performance, effect on 150, 159

Index

Index

Index

Index

Index

Index

Index

Index

Index

Index

Index

Index

Index

Index